Early Nutrition Programming and Health Outcomes in Later Life

Obesity and Beyond

Berthold Koletzko • Tamás Decsi
Dénes Molnár • Anne de la Hunty
Editors

Early Nutrition Programming and Health Outcomes in Later Life

Obesity and Beyond

Springer

Editors
Berthold Koletzko
Coordinator
The Early Nutrition Programming Project
and
Professor of Paediatrics
Dr. von Hauner Children's Hospital
University of Munich
Germany

Tamás Decsi
Professor of Paediatrics
Department of Paediatrics
University of Pécs
József A. u. 7., Pécs, 7623
Hungary

Dénes Molnár
Professor of Paediatrics
Department of Paediatrics
University of Pécs
József A. u. 7., Pécs, 7623
Hungary

Anne de la Hunty
Ashwell Associates (Europe) Ltd.
Ashwell Street, Ashwell
Hertfordshire, SG7 5PZ
UK

ISBN 978-94-017-7713-1 ISBN 978-1-4020-9173-5 (eBook)
DOI 10.1007/978-1-4020-9173-5

Softcover re-print of the Hardcover 1st edition 2009

Printed on acid-free paper

springer.com

Preface

At first, the evidence for early nutrition programming in humans, with its emphasis on low birth weight babies and fetal growth restriction, suggested that the concept might have only a limited application to a small group of the population. It appeared unable to offer any remedies for current health problems such as the dramatic increase in the prevalence of obesity and its consequences. More recently however, the observation that fetal overnutrition may lead to the same outcomes as fetal undernutrition in terms of increased risk of obesity, hypertension, insulin resistance and CVD in adult life, implied that programming effects are seen across the nutritional spectrum and this has lead to the search for a common mechanism. The role of accelerated growth, either due to catch-up growth after fetal growth restriction or to faster growth rates in formula fed infants has been suggested as a unifying factor and is one possible common mechanism which is being investigated. Furthermore, the possibility that maternal obesity might programme fetal growth and metabolism to be more susceptible to weight gain in later life gives rise to the potential for an intergenerational cycle of obesity which can only make matters worse. These insights have greatly extended the scope and potential impact of the early nutrition programming concept and have shown that it is of huge contemporary relevance with major public health significance.

This volume contains recent findings presented at the International Conference on Early Nutrition Programming and Health Outcomes in Later Life: Obesity and Beyond – a satellite meeting of the 15th European Congress on Obesity, held in Budapest in April 2007. Basic scientific research, data from epidemiological studies and clinical trial results were all presented during the programme. This volume includes articles discussing the evidence for an effect of early nutrition programming on later obesity and cardiovascular risk; the growing evidence for an intergenerational cycle of obesity; the role of maternal leptin in programming appetite; possible cellular mechanisms for altered energy balance, including mitochondrial programming and the effects of regulators of metabolism; and how epigenetic changes might be the fundamental underlying mechanism explaining programming effects. Consumer understanding of the concept of early nutrition programming and the extent to which early nutrition programming is taken into account in infant feeding policies are also discussed.

The conference attracted more than 250 scientists from over 30 countries around the world. European scientists were well represented but there were also many participants from outside the EU including the US, Australia and New Zealand, Japan, the Middle East and Russia. The conference was a joint meeting between the Early Nutrition Programming Project and the European Academy of Nutritional Sciences and was organised by the University of Munich, Germany and the University of Pécs, Hungary. We are very grateful to the Directorate General Research of the European Commission which provided major financial support to hold the conference, and also to Martek Biosciences Corporation, the Nestlé Research Centre, Merck Darmstadt and DSM Nutritional Products Ltd for their generous co-sponsorship of the meeting, as well as to Ordesa and Novalac United Pharmaceuticals for their sponsorship of Young Investigators travel grants. We would also like to thank Professor Peter Aggett, the president of the European Academy of Nutritional Sciences, and the members of the scientific committee for their help in developing the scientific programme; the conference speakers for their thoughtful contributions; Dr. Hans Demmelmair and Dr. Julia von Rosen for their efficient organising of the conference; Dr. Margaret Ashwell and Rhonda Smith for their effective dissemination of the conference information; Anne de la Hunty for editing these proceedings and Isabelle de Froidmont-Görtz from the EC Directorate General Research for her sympathetic support for the Early Nutrition Programming Project.

It is our hope that these proceedings will help stimulate further progress in research and lead to improved nutrition policies for reversing the current rise in obesity levels in Europe.

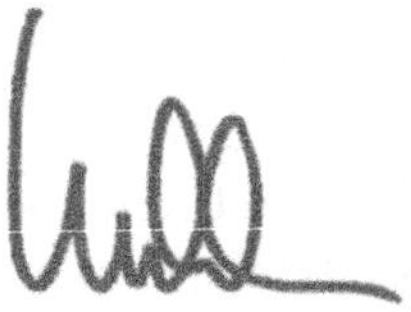

Berthold Koletzko, MD
Professor of Paediatrics, University of Munich
Coordinator, The Early Nutrition Programming Project
(www.metabolic-programming.org)

Contents

Challenges and Novel Approaches in the Epidemiological Study of Early Life Influences on Later Disease

George Davey Smith, Sam Leary, Andy Ness, and Debbie A. Lawlor

Abstract The influence of factors acting during early life on health outcomes of offspring is of considerable research and public health interest. There are, however, methodological challenges in establishing robust causal links, since exposures often act many decades before outcomes of interest, and may also be strongly related to other factors, generating considerable degrees of potential confounding. With respect to pre-natal factors, the degree of counfounding can sometimes be estimated by comparing the association between exposures experienced by the mother during pregnancy and outcomes among the offspring with the association of the same exposures experienced by the father during the pregnancy period and offspring outcomes. If the effects are due to an intra-uterine exposure, then maternal exposure during pregnancy should have a clearly greater influence than paternal exposure. If confounding by socio-economic, behavioural or genetic factors generates the association then maternal and paternal pregnancy exposures will be related in the same way with the outcome. For early life exposures it is also possible to compare outcomes in siblings who are concordant or discordant for the exposure, which will reduce the influence of family-level confounding factors. A different approach is that of Mendelian randomization, which utilises genetic variants of known effect that can proxy for modifiable exposures and are also not in general related to potential confounding factors, or influenced by disease. In other settings the use of non-genetic instrumental variables is possible. A series of examples of the application of these approaches are presented and their potentials and limitations discussed. Other epidemiological strategies are briefly reviewed.

G. Davey Smith(✉)
Department of Social Medicine, University of Bristol, Canynge Hall,
Whiteladies Road, Bristol BS8 2PR
george.davey-smith@bristol.ac.uk

G. Davey Smith and D.A. Lawlor
MRC Centre for Causal Analyses in Translational Epidemiology, University of Bristol,
Canynge Hall, Whiteladies Road, Bristol BS8 2PR

S. Leary and A. Ness
Department of Oral and Dental Science, University of Bristol,
Lower Maudlin Street, Bristol BS1 2LY

B. Koletzko et al. (eds.), *Early Nutrition Programming and Health Outcomes in Later Life: Obesity and Beyond*,

It is concluded that the naïve acceptance of findings utilising conventional epidemiological methods in this setting is misplaced.

Keywords Causal inference • developmental origins • family studies • Mendelian randomization

Abbreviations ALSPAC: Avon Longitudinal Study of Parents and their Children; BMI: body mass index; IV: instrumental variable; MTHFR: methyltetrahydrofolate reductase; NTD: neural tube defects; RCT: randomised controlled trials

1 Introduction

There is considerable interest in the proposition that exposures acting in early life have long-term consequences for health in adulthood. The early life factors include those acting during (or before) the period of fetal development – such as maternal diet, smoking or alcohol use; those acting in infancy – such as breast or bottle feeding; and those acting in childhood – such as passive exposure to tobacco smoke. Nearly all domains of later health experience – including cardiovascular disease, various cancers, respiratory disease and cognitive decline – have been associated with early-life exposures of one kind or another. To formulate effective public health policy it is crucial to be able to separate out causal associations, which offer the possibility of intervention and disease prevention, from non-causal associations. If the non-causal associations are mistaken for causal associations this could lead to misguided strategies that at best waste resources and divert attention from effective approaches, and at worst could have health-damaging consequences.

2 Challenges Facing Epidemiological Studies of Early Life Influences

There are several issues that render the epidemiological study of the influence of early life exposures on later health outcomes problematic. These relate to the long time-gap between exposure and outcome. The assessment of exposure may be difficult, since retrospective approaches may be required to obtain information regarding exposures acting many decades before the health outcome is observed. There are no truly prospective large-scale studies with detailed and continuous data – including biological measures – from before birth through to late adulthood. Such problematic exposure assessment can lead to random errors, with the expectation that these errors would attenuate effect estimates and make it more difficult to establish robust associations. This will lead to studies being underpowered, but not to spurious associations being observed. Perhaps more seriously retrospective assessment may be biased by knowledge of later health outcomes. Biased exposure reporting can, in this situation, generate spurious associations when none actually exist.

A further consequence of the long time gap between exposure and outcome is that even when associations are observed from well-conducted prospective studies, and therefore likely to be robust, their relevance to contemporary pregnant women, infants and children is unclear. Thus findings in lifecourse epidemiology may be context dependent, and long time gaps between exposure and outcome render it more likely that they will not be applicable to current exposure patterns.

A further challenge to causal inference is the potential for substantial degrees of confounding. For example, a number of studies have investigated the effect of breast feeding on later health outcomes, such as obesity, blood pressure, cancer risk and cognitive function. However in many societies breast feeding is strongly related to higher socioeconomic circumstances and associated phenomena, such as maternal non-smoking, healthy diet, low toxic occupational exposures and a generally better quality of the physical and social environment. The links between breast feeding and these other factors would generate relationships between breast feeding and the many health outcomes that they influence. Thus it has been claimed that the association between breast feeding and IQ can be completely accounted for by such confounding (Der et al. 2006).

3 Examples of Mismatch Between Observational and Trial Evidence

Confounding and bias are capable of generating associations in observational epidemiological studies of adulthood risk factors and disease outcomes that are not causal. Consider cardiovascular disease, where observational studies suggesting that beta carotene, (Manson et al. 1991) vitamin E supplements, (Rimm et al. 1993; Stampfer et al. 1993) vitamin C supplements, (Osganian et al. 2003) and hormone replacement therapy (HRT) (Stampfer and Colditz 1991) were protective were followed by large randomised controlled trials (RCT) showing no such protection. (Omenn et al. 1996; Alpha-tocopherol 1994; Dietary supplementation 1999; Heart Protection Study 2002; Beral et al. 2002; Manson et al. 2003). In each case special pleading was advanced to explain the discrepancy, but it is likely that a general problem of confounding – by lifestyle and socioeconomic factors, or by baseline health status and prescription policies – is responsible (Davey Smith and Ebrahim 2001, 2006; Lawlor et al. 2004; Vandenbroucke 2004).

There is evidence that the intake or level of antioxidants is associated with known risk factors for coronary heart disease. In the British Women's Heart and Health study (BWHHS), for example, women with higher plasma vitamin C levels were less likely to be in a manual social class, have no car access, be a smoker or be obese and more likely to exercise, be on a low fat diet, have a daily alcoholic drink, and be tall (Lawlor et al. 2004, 2005a). Furthermore for these women in their 60s and 70s, those with higher plasma vitamin C levels were less likely to have come from a home 50 years or more previously in which their father was in a manual job, or had no bathroom or hot water, or within which they had to share a bedroom. They were also less likely to have limited educational attainment. In short, a substantial amount of confounding by factors from across the lifecourse that predict elevated risk of coronary heart disease was seen.

There are similar instances of confounding and bias operating in studies of early-life factors and later health outcomes. Consider, for example, the influence of maternal diet on offspring health and development. In the Southampton Women's Study there are very strong associations between diet, socio-economic position and smoking. (Robinson et al. 2004). In observational studies vitamin C intake during pregnancy has been associated with higher birth weight of offspring (Matthews et al. 1999), however data such as those from Robinson et al. (2004) would suggest that mothers with higher vitamin C intake during pregnancy would have much lower rates of smoking and be of more privileged socio-economic background, generating substantial confounding. Figure 1 contrasts the results from the observational study with those from the largest RCT to date in which pregnant women were randomised to a supplement containing vitamin C and E (Poston et al. 2006). Findings from the two study designs are unlikely to be compatible.

Given the inherent difficulties in relating early life exposures to later health outcomes, in this chapter we will briefly discuss several methods that can be applied

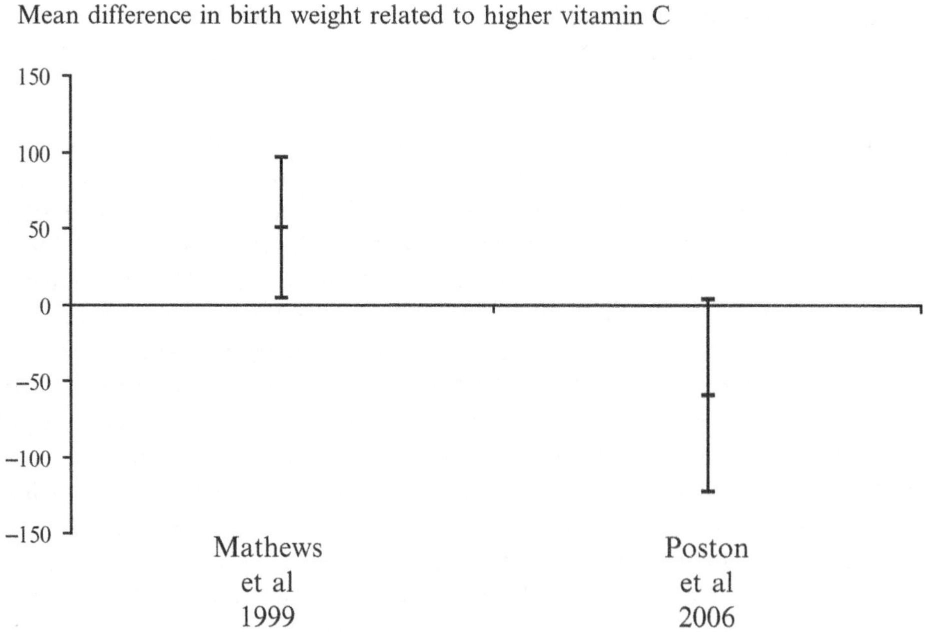

Fig. 1 Comparison of observational epidemiological evidence and randomised controlled trial evidence of the association between maternal vitamin C intake during pregnancy and birth weight

in epidemiological studies to increase the ability to draw causal inferences. These approaches include the use of maternal/paternal comparisons, studies of siblings, the identification of critical time periods and the use of genetic and non-genetic instrumental variable approaches. The approaches described here constitute a far from exhaustive list, but we hope illustrate methods that have some general utility.

4 Contrasting Maternal and Paternal Exposure Associations with Offspring Outcomes

We are often interested in the possibility that maternal exposures during pregnancy have a direct biological effect on offspring outcomes, through influencing the intrauterine environment in which the fetal development of the offspring occurs. Thus maternal smoking may influence offspring obesity, or maternal alcohol use may lead to impairments in various aspects of offspring functioning. However there are many confounding factors that could generate non-causal links between the smoking and drinking behaviours of mothers and the health of their children. One approach to this issue is to compare the strength of associations between an exposure among mothers and offspring outcomes with the association between the same exposure among fathers and the offspring outcomes (Davey Smith 2008). If there were a direct biological effect of intrauterine exposure on offspring health status, then the link with offspring health should be much stronger for exposure among mothers than for exposure among fathers. This can be illustrated with respect to an outcome where there is strong evidence of a causal influence of a maternal exposure – maternal smoking during pregnancy and on offspring health outcome, birthweight. Figure 2 demonstrates that in the Avon Longitudinal Study of Parents and their Children (ALSPAC) maternal smoking during pregnancy is associated with lower offspring birthweight, whereas smoking by the

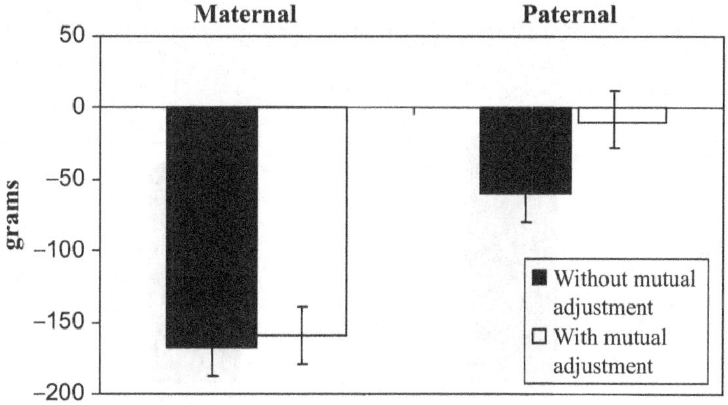

Fig. 2 Association between maternal/paternal smoking and offspring birthweight without and with mutual adjustment (difference in birthweight between offspring whose parents are smokers and non-smokers in grams)

father during pregnancy is only weakly associated (presumably because of some confounding with maternal smoking), and when both maternal and paternal smoking during pregnancy are taken into account the former shows a robust association that is little attenuated, whereas the latter association is essentially abolished.

There has been considerable interest in the possibility that maternal smoking influences fetal development in a way that leads to higher body mass index (BMI) and risk of obesity in later life. In the case of offspring BMI at age 7 initial examination of the ALSPAC data show that the average BMI of children of smoking mothers is raised (Fig. 3; Leary et al. 2006a). However a similar sized association is seen with smoking by fathers, and including both maternal and paternal smoking behaviour in the same model leaves residual effects of similar magnitude (Fig. 3). These findings suggest, that in the case of offspring BMI, maternal smoking during pregnancy does not have a direct intrauterine effect, rather confounding factors associated with parental smoking and offspring BMI generate an association between both maternal and paternal smoking and offspring BMI. By contrast, for offspring leg length at age 7, maternal smoking shows stronger effects than paternal smoking (Leary et al. 2006b), suggesting a biological effect of maternal smoking on femur development, as supported by other studies of this issue (Jaddoe et al. 2007).

In our view, the strong implication of finding that maternal and paternal lifestyle-related factors during pregnancy are associated in similar ways with offspring outcomes suggests that such associations are generated by underlying socially-patterned environmental influences acting at the family level, and do not reflect direct biological influences of the exposures *per se*. However it is possible to interpret the findings differently. For example Pembrey et al. (2006) suggest that the association between paternal smoking and offspring BMI reflects epigenetic influences, and that such male-line transgenerational responses have important health implications. While it is possible that these male-line epigenetic factors exactly match the biological influence of maternal smoking on the intrauterine environment, to generate very similar associations, we feel this is unlikely. Informal or formal approaches to comparing explanatory models,

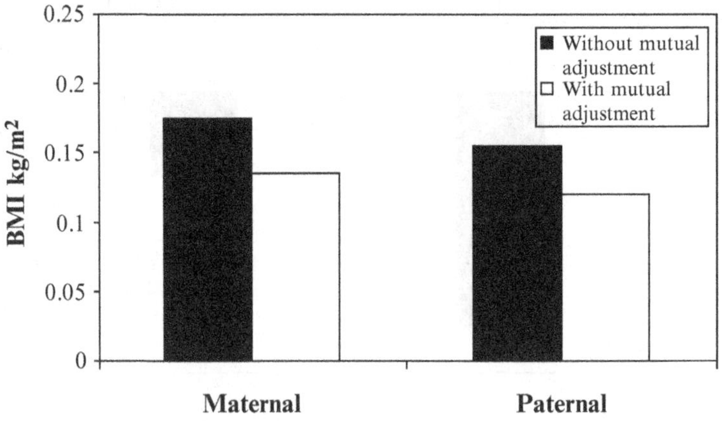

Fig. 3 Effect of maternal and paternal smoking during pregnancy on offspring body mass index without and with mutual adjustment

which adopt the parsimony principle of Occam's Razor (i.e. making the fewest possible assumptions) (Mackay 2003), would suggest that the likelihood of such perfectly matched effects, being produced by mechanistically distinct processes, is rather low.

5 Within and Between Sibship Comparisons

As we discuss above there are many factors that can confound associations between early life influences and later outcomes. One approach to this that has been widely utilised in the social sciences is to compare associations within sibling pairs and between all the people in a study, independent of their sibling group (Conley et al. 2003). Since familial socioeconomic background will be similar for siblings from the same family, comparing outcome differences in relation to discordant exposure levels within sibships is in effect 'matching' on fixed family characteristics (including socioeconomic position), whether these are evaluated or not in a study. As such this provides a stronger means of controlling for family socioeconomic position than multivariable adjustment, particularly where studies only have one or two indicators of socioeconomic position.

Consider, for example, the influence of breastfeeding on later growth. We know that in many situations breast-feeding is strongly socially patterned, and will be related to a whole series of factors that might lead to greater growth amongst people who are breast fed. In a prospective cohort study of 4,999 children from 1,352 families born in the 1920s and 1930s, breast feeding was related to later growth (Martin et al. 2002). When the analyses were undertaken in the whole cohort with no attention to within sibship associations, breast fed subjects were taller in childhood than never breast fed subjects. The association between breast feeding and childhood height and leg length persisted when the analysis was restricted to within sibship height/leg length differences in relation to within sibship differences in breast feeding. These findings were interpreted as demonstrating that breast feeding is causally related to greater skeletal growth (i.e. that the association is not confounded by fixed familial effects such as socioeconomic background). RCT evidence suggests that exclusive breast feeding results in accelerated growth in the first few months of life, but with no detectable difference by 12 months (effects on later childhood height have yet to be reported) (Kramer et al. 2002). However, the issue of context dependence discussed above may well apply here, as the food received by non-breast fed infants in the 1920s and 1930s in the U.K. will be very different to that received by the infants in the RCT, carried out in Belarus in the late 1990s.

Authors of studies that have compared within and between sibship associations point out that these studies provide insights into potential mechanisms between exposures and outcomes found in general population studies, beyond simply determining whether these are due to confounding or not (Lawlor et al. 2006b, 2007a). These comparisons require careful consideration of factors that are the same for siblings brought-up together. Thus, in a very large Swedish record linkage study inverse associations of birth weight and gestational age with systolic blood pressure were found both within and between sibships (Lawlor et al. 2007). These findings suggest that the association between birth weight or gestational age and systolic blood pressure are not explained by factors, such as family socioeconomic position, that are the same or very similar for siblings. With additional intergenerational data included in the analyses the authors concluded that intrauterine factors, such as the effects of maternal metabolic or vascular health during pregnancy and/or placental function (characteristics that will vary from one pregnancy to the next in the same mother) were the most likely explanation for the association of birth weight/ gestational age with blood pressure in the general population.

Several authors have used within and between sibling studies to explore whether the consistent positive association between birth weight and later intelligence (Lawlor et al. 2006a) is due to confounding or not (Record et al. 1969; Matte et al. 2001; Lawlor et al. 2005b, 2006c). These studies have produced discrepant findings, with some (e.g. Lawlor et al. 2005b; Matte et al. 2001) suggesting that birth weight discrepancies within sibships are related to differences in intelligence, and others (e.g. Lawlor et al. 2006c; Record et al. 1969) finding no such association. As two (Record et al. 1969; Lawlor et al. 2006c) of the largest studies found no within sibship association, and the third large study found a within sibship effect only for a sub-group (that was not clearly pre-specified) of males only (Matte et al. 2001) – it therefore seems reasonable to conclude that the association between birth weight and childhood intelligence seen in general populations of singletons is largely explained by factors, such as family socioeconomic background and parental education, that are shared by siblings. These studies demonstrate the need for large sample sizes if robust evidence is to be obtained from within and between sibship studies.

6 Relating an Exposure to a Critical Period

In some cases an exposure only influences a disease outcome if experienced during a critical exposure window. However confounding factors or biases would generally generate associations between exposure at any time and the outcome. Thus demonstrating the specific influence of an exposure at a particular critical window and a health outcome provides some evidence that the association is causal. For example, it has been suggested that radiotherapy for Hodgkin's lymphoma increases the later risk of breast cancer. However many factors could generate an association between Hodgkin's lymphoma and breast cancer. Such confounding factors would, however, apply to Hodgkin's lymphoma diagnosed at any stage of life. Thus the demonstration that exposure to radiotherapy for Hodgkin's lymphoma between menarche and first pregnancy – when the breast is particularly sensitive to mitogens – but not at other times is related to increased risk of breast cancer many years later provides some evidence that this is a causal association. That said, these analyses need to be pre-specified and those that are not should be clearly identified as post-hoc exploratory analyses that require confirmation.

7 Mendelian Randomisation

Mendelian randomization is the term that has been given to studies that use genetic variants in observational epidemiology to make causal inferences about modifiable (non-genetic) risk factors for disease and health related outcomes (Youngman et al. 2000; Davey Smith and Ebrahim 2003; Davey Smith 2007). Such studies exploit what is known as Mendel's second law or the law of independent assortment:

> *that the behavior of each pair of differentiating characters in hybrid union is independent of the other differences between the two original plants, and, further, that the hybrid produces just so many kinds of* egg *and pollen cells as there are possible constant combination forms.* (Mendel 1865)

In simple terms this means that the inheritance of one trait is independent of (i.e. randomised with respect to) the inheritance of other traits. The independent distribution of alleles (or blocks of alleles in linkage disequilibrium) from parents to their offspring means that a study relating health outcomes in the offspring to genetic variation transmitted from the parents will not suffer from confounding. This holds true for full-siblings who are not monozygotic twins. Despite the actual random allocation of groups of alleles being at the level of parent to offspring dyads, at a population level – when relating genetic variants to disease outcome – alleles are generally unrelated to those confounding factors (in particular socioeconomic position and lifestyle factors) that distort the interpretations of findings from observational epidemiology (Bhatti et al. 2005; Davey Smith et al. 2008). Furthermore, disease processes do not alter germline genotype and therefore associations between genotype and disease outcomes cannot be affected by reverse causality. Finally, for genetic variants that are related to a modifiable exposure this will generally be the case throughout life from birth to adulthood and therefore their use in causal inference can also avoid attenuation by errors (regression dilution bias) (Davey Smith and Ebrahim 2004), and provides an estimate of the effect of a modifiable exposure across the life course on disease outcome (Kivimaki et al. 2007). Mendelian randomization studies have been likened to a 'natural' RCT (Davey Smith and Ebrahim 2005; Hingorani and Humphries 2005). In addition to the major advantages with respect to confounding, unlike with conventional RCTs, Mendelian randomization studies can be conducted in a representative population sample without the need for exclusion criteria or for volunteers amenable to being randomly allocated to treatment.

Mendelian Randomization studies can provide unique insights into the causal nature of early life effects on later disease outcomes. For example, it is now widely accepted that neural tube defects (NTDs) can in part be prevented by periconceptual maternal folate supplementation (Scholl and Johnson 2000). RCTs of folate supplementation have provided the key evidence in this regard (MRC Vitamin Study 1991; Czeizel and Dudás 1992). But could we have reached the same conclusion before the RCTs were carried out, if we had access to evidence from genetic association studies? Studies have been carried out that have looked at the MTHFR 677C→T polymorphism (a genetic variant that is associated with methyltetrahydrofolate reductase activity and circulating folate and homocysteine levels; the TT genotype being associated with lower circulating folate levels) in newborns with NTDs compared to controls, and have found an increased risk in TT versus CC newborns, with a relative risk of 1.75 (95% CI 1.41–2.18) in a meta-analysis of all such studies (Botto and Yang 2000). Studies have also looked at the association between this MTHFR variant in parents and the risk of NTD in their offspring. Mothers who have the TT genotype have an increased risk of 2.04 (95% CI 1.49–2.81) of having an offspring with a NTD compared to mothers who have the CC genotype (Botto and Yang 2000). For TT fathers, the equivalent relative risk is 1.18 (95% CI 0.65–2.12) (Botto and Yang 2000). This pattern of associations suggests that it is the intra-uterine environment – influenced by maternal TT genotype – rather than the genotype of offspring that is related to disease risk (Fig. 4). This is consistent with the hypothesis that maternal folate intake is the exposure of importance.

In this case the findings from observational studies, genetic associations studies and an RCT are similar. Had the technology been available, the genetic association studies, with the particular influence of maternal versus paternal genotype on NTD risk, would have provided evidence of the beneficial effect of folate supplementation before the results of any RCT had been completed. Certainly, the genetic association studies would have provided better evidence than that given by conventional epidemiological studies that had to cope with the problems of accurately assessing diet and also with the considerable confounding of maternal folate intake with a wide variety of lifestyle and socioeconomic factors that may also influence NTD risk. The association of genotype with NTD risk does not suggest that genetic screening is indicated – rather it demonstrates that an environmental intervention may benefit the whole population, independent of the genotype of individuals receiving intervention. There are an increasing number of examples in which Mendelian randomization can be utilized to understand the causal nature of intra-uterine exposures, the major (but diminishing) limitations being the identification of genetic variants that are robustly associated with environmentally-modifiable

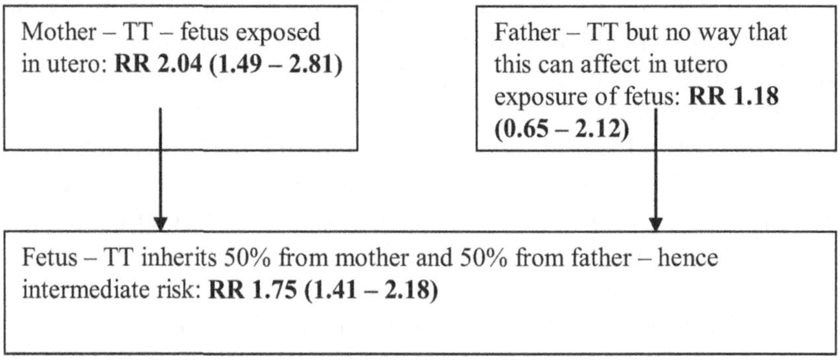

Fig. 4 Inheritance of MTHFR polymorphism, homocysteine and neural tube defects

risk processes and the size of the studies required to provide robust estimates of the association.

8 Non-genetic Instrumental Variables

The use of genotype, in Mendelian randomisation studies, to provide causal inference for the effect of a modifiable (non-genetic) exposure on disease outcome is an application of the general theory of *instrumental variables analysis* (Lawlor et al. 2008). An *instrumental variable* (IV) is a variable that is associated with the outcome only through its robust association with the exposure of interest. As such an instrumental variable will not be associated with factors that confound the association of exposure with outcome.

Dehydration in infancy has been associated with increased later blood pressure in one small study (Davey Smith et al. 2006). Furthermore a potential mechanism exists through a predictive adaptive response relating to the selective advantage of being able to respond to one episode of severe dehydration by sodium retention. However dehydration early in life will be strongly confounded with later-life exposures. One study interested in whether dehydration during early infancy was a risk factor for higher blood pressure later in life used climate conditions during infancy as an instrumental variable for the effect of dehydration (Lawlor et al. 2006d). Severe dehydration in early infancy might programme a taste for salty food in later life, which could result in greater blood pressure (Fessler 2003). Testing this hypothesis is problematic both because any assessment of dehydration in early life is difficult and the likelihood of an infant being dehydrated will be related to a number of socioeconomic and lifestyle confounding factors.

Rates of infant mortality and morbidity from diarrhoeal illnesses increased considerably during the summer months in the early decades of the twentieth century in Britain (Lawlor et al. 2006d). This summer diarrhoea and its associated infant mortality occurred in epidemic proportions during the hottest and driest (compared to cooler and wetter) summers. Thus, adults who were born in the early part of the last century and who experienced hot dry summers during the first year of their life are more likely than those who experienced cooler and wetter summers to have suffered infant diarrhoea and dehydration. Climate conditions in infancy for such a population would be a valid instrumental variable since there is no reason for it to be associated with socioeconomic and lifestyle confounding factors, as found amongst participants in the British Women's Heart and Health Study, a random sample of 3,964 British women born in the 1920s and 1930s. However, a one standard deviation (1.3°C) higher mean summer temperature in the first year of life was associated with a 1.12 mmHg (95% CI: 0.33, 1.91 mmHg) higher adult systolic blood pressure, and a one standard deviation higher mean summer rainfall (33.9 mm) with a lower systolic blood pressure (–1.65 [–2.44, –0.85] mmHg) (Lawlor et al. 2006d).

9 Conclusions

We have discussed various approaches to increasing the strength of causal inference in studies of early life exposure and later health outcomes. They have one characteristic in common, and that is that they generally require large sample sizes. This is because some of the methods require formal statistical tests between the strength of different associations (between maternal and paternal effects, for example), and others relate to situations of known small effect size (such as the association between common genetic variants and disease outcomes in the case of Mendelian randomization). However the price of large sample sizes is certainly one worth paying to get closer to reliable estimates of causal effects in epidemiological studies.

Acknowledgements Debbie Lawlor is funded by a UK Department of Health Career Scientist Award.

References

Alpha-Tocopherol, Beta Carotene Cancer Prevention Study Group (1994). The effect of vitamin E and beta carotene on the incidence of lung cancer and other cancers in male smokers. *N Engl J Med* **330**: 1029–1035.

Beral V, Banks E, Reeves G (2002). Evidence from randomized trials of the long-term effects of hormone replacement therapy. *Lancet* **360**: 942–944.

Bhatti P, Sigurdson AJ, Wang SS, Chen J, Rothman N, Hartge P, Bergen AW, Landi MT (2005). Genetic variation and willingness to participate in epidemiologic research: data from three studies. *Cancer Epidemiol Biomar Prev* **14**: 2449–2453.

Botto LD, Yang Q (2000). 5, 10-Methylenetetrahydrofolate reductase gene variants and congenital anomalies: a HuGE Review. *Am J Epidemiol* **151**: 862–877.

Conley D, Strully KW, Bennett NG (2003). *The starting gate. Birth weight and life chances.* Berkeley, CA: University of California Press.

Czeizel AE, Dudás I (1992). Prevention of the first occurrence of neural-tube defects by periconceptional vitamin supplementation. *New Engl J Med* **327**: 1832–1835.

Davey Smith G (2000). Capitalising on Mendelian randomisation to assess the effects of treatment. *J. Royal Soc Med* **100**: 432–435.

Davey Smith G (2008). Assessing intrauterine influences on offspring health outcomes: can epidemiological findings yield robust results? *Basic Clini Pharmacol Toxicol* **102**: 245–256.

Davey Smith G, Ebrahim S (2001). Epidemiology: is it time to call it a day? *Int J Epidemiol* **30**: 1–14.

Davey Smith G, Ebrahim S (2003). "Mendelian randomisation": can genetic epidemiology contribute to understanding environmental determinants of disease? *Int J Epidemiol* **32**: 1–22.

Davey Smith G, Ebrahim S (2004). Mendelian randomization: prospects, potentials, and limitations. *Int J Epidemiol* **33**: 30–42.

Davey Smith G, Ebrahim S (2005) What can Mendelian randomisation tell us about modifiable behavioural and environmental exposures. *BMJ*; **330**: 1076–1079.

Davey Smith G, Ebrahim S (2006). Folate supplementation and cardiovascular disease. *Lancet* **366**: 1679–1681.

Davey Smith G, Leary S, Ness A (2006). Dehyration in infancy and later blood pressure. *J Epidemiol Community Health* **60**: 142–143.

Davey Smith G, Lawlor DA, Harbord R, Timpson N, Day I, Ebrahim S (2008). Clustered environments and randomized genes: a fundamental distinction between conventional and genetic epidemiology. *PloS Med* **4**: 1985–1992.

Der G, Batty GD, Deary IJ (2006). Effect of breast feeding on intelligence in children: prospective study, sibling pairs analysis, and meta-analysis. *Brit Med J* **333**: 945.

Dietary supplementation (1999). With n-3 polyunsaturated fatty acids and vitamin E after myocardial infarction: results of the GISSI-Prevenzione trial. Gruppo Italiano per lo Studio della Sopravvivenza nell'Infarto miocardico. *Lancet* **354**: 447–455.

Fessler DM (2003). An evolutionary explanation of the plasticity of salt preferences: prophylaxis against sudden dehydration. *Med Hypotheses* **61**: 412–415.

Heart Protection Study Collaborative Group (2002). MRC/BHF Heart Protection Study of antioxidant vitamin supplementation in 20536 high-risk individuals: a randomised placebo-controlled trial. *Lancet* **360**: 23–33.

Hingorani A, Humphries S (2005). Nature's randomised trials. *Lancet* **366**: 1906–1908.

Jaddoe VWV, Berburg BE, de Ridder MAJ, Hofman A, Mackenbach JP, Moll HA, Steegers EAP, Witteman JCM (2007). Maternal smoking and fetal growth characteristics in different periods of pregnancy. *Am J Epidemiol* **165**: 1207–1215.

Kivimaki M, Lawlor DA, Davey Smith G, Eklund C, Hurme M, Lehtimaki T et al. (2007). Variants in the CRP gene as a measure of life-long differences in average C-reactive protein levels: the cardiovascular risk in Young Finns Study. *Am J Epidemiol* **166**: 760–764.

Kramer MS, Guo T, Platt RW, Shapiro S, Collet JP, Chalmers B et al. (2002). Breastfeeding and infant growth: biology or bias? *Pediatrics* **110**(2 Pt 1): 343–347.

Lawlor DA, Davey Smith G, Bruckdorfer KR et al. (2004). Those confounded vitamins: what can we learn from the differences between observational versus randomised trial evidence? *Lancet* **363**: 1724–1727.

Lawlor DA, Ebrahim S, Kundu D, Bruckdorfer KR, Whincup PH, Davey Smith G (2005a). Vitamin C is not associated with coronary heart disease risk once life course socioeconomic position is taken into account: prospective findings from the British Women's Heart and Health Study. *Heart* **91**: 1086–1087.

Lawlor DA, Bor W, O'Callaghan MJ, Williams GM, Najman JM (2005b). Intrauterine growth and intelligence within sibling pairs: findings from the Mater-University study of pregnancy and its outcomes. *J Epidemiol Community Health* **59**: 279–282.

Lawlor DA, Najman JM, Batty GD, C'Callaghan MJ, Williams GM, Bor W (2006a). Early life predictors of childhood intelligence: findings from the Mater-University study of pregnancy and its outcomes. *Paediatr Perinat Epidemiol* **20**: 148–162.

Lawlor DA, Clark H, Davey Smith G, Leon DA (2006b). Childhood intelligence, educational attainment and adult body mass index: findings from a prospective cohort and within sibling-pairs analysis. *Int J Obes* **30**: 1758–1765.

Lawlor DA, Clark H, Davey Smith G, Leon DA (2006c). Intrauterine growth and intelligence within sibling-pairs: findings from the Aberdeen Children of the 1950s cohort. *Pediatrics* 117:e894–e902.

Lawlor DA, Davey Smith G, Mitchell R, Ebrahim S (2006d). Adult blood pressure and climate conditions in infancy: a test of the hypothesis that dehydration in infancy increases adult blood pressure. *Am J Epidemiol* **163**: 608–614.

Lawlor DA, Hübinette A, Tynelius P, Leon DA, Davey Smith G, Rasmussen F (2007a). The associations of gestational age and intrauterine growth with systolic blood pressure in a family based study of 386,485 men in 331,089 families. *Circulation* **115**: 562–568.

Lawlor DA, Harbord RM, Sterne JAC, Timpson N, Davey Smith G (2007b). Mendelian randomization: using genes as instruments for making causal inferences in epidemiology. *Stat Med* **27**: 1133–1163.

Leary S, Davey Smith G, Ness A, ALSPAC Study team (2006a). Smoking during pregnancy and components of stature in the offspring. *Am J Hum Biol* **18**: 502–512.

Leary SD, Davey Smith G, Rogers IS, Reilly JJ, Wells JCK, Ness AR (2006b). Smoking during pregnancy and offspring fat and lean mass in childhood. *Obesity* **14**: 2284–2293.

Mackay DJ (2003). Model comparison and Occams Razor. In: Mackay DJ (ed.), *Information theory, inference and learning algorithms*. Cambridge: Cambridge University Press.
Manson J, Stampfer MJ, Willett WC, Colditz G, Rosner B, Speizer FE, Hennekens CH (1991). A prospective study of antioxidant vitamins and incidence of coronary heart disease in women. *Circulation* **84**(Suppl II): II-546.
Manson JE, Hsia J, Johnson KC et al. (2003) Estrogen plus progestin and the risk of coronary heart disease. *NEJM* **349**: 523–534.
Martin RM, Davey Smith G, Mangtani P, Frankel S, Gunnell D (2002). Association between breastfeeding and growth: the Boyd Orr cohort study. *Arch Dis Child* **87**: F193–F201.
Matte TD, Bresnahan M, Begg MD, Susser E (2001, Aug 11). Influence of variation in birth weight within normal range and within sibships on IQ at age 7 years: cohort study. *BMJ* **323**(7308): 310–314. Erratum in: *BMJ* 2001, Sep 22; **323**(7314): 684.
Matthews F, Yudkin P, Neil A (1999). Influence of maternal nutrition on outcome of pregnancy: prospective cohort study. *BMJ* **319**: 339–343.
Mendel, G (1865). Experiments in plant hybridization. http://www.mendelweb.org/archive/Mendel.Experiments.txt. Accessed May 2007.
MRC Vitamin Study Research Group (1991). Prevention of neural tube defects: results of the Medical Research Council vitamin study. *Lancet* **338**: 131–137.
Omenn GS, Goodman GE, Thornquist MD et al. (1996). Effects of a combination of beta carotene and vitamin A on lung cancer and cardiovascular disease. *N Engl J Med* **334**: 1150–1155.
Osganian SK, Stampfer MJ, Rimm E, Spiegelman D, Hu FB, Manson JE, Willett WC (2003). Vitamin C and risk of coronary heart disease in women. *J Am Coll Cardiol* **42**: 246–252.
Pembrey ME, Bygren LO, Kaati G, Edvinsson S, Northstone K, Sjöström M, Golding J, ALSPAC Study Team (2006). Sex-specific, male-line transgenerational responses in humans. *Eur J Hum Genet* **14**: 159–166.
Poston L, Briley AL, Seed PT, Kelly FJ, Sheenan, for the Vitamins in Pre-eclampsia (VIP) Trial Consortium (2006). Vitamin C and vitamin E in pregnant women at risk for pre-eclampsia (VIP trial): randomised placebo-controlled trial. *Lancet* **367**: 1145.
Record RG, McKeown T, Edwards JH (1969). The relation of measured intelligence to birth weight and duration of gestation. *Ann Hum Genet* **33**: 71–79.
Rimm EB, Stampfer MJ, Ascherio A, Giovannucci E, Colditz GA, Willett WC (1993). Vitamin E consumption and the risk of coronary heart disease in men. *New Engl J Med* **328**: 1450–1456.
Robinson SM, Crozier SR, Borland SE, Hammond J, Barker DJP, Inskip HM (2004). Impact of educational attainment on the quality of young women's diets. *Eur J Clin Nutr* **158**: 1174–1180.
Scholl TO, Johnson WG (2000). Folic acid: influence on the outcome of pregnancy. *Am J Clin Nutr* **71**(Suppl): 1295S–1303S.
Stampfer MJ, Colditz GA (1991). Estrogen replacement therapy and coronary heart disease: a quantitative assessment of the epidemiologic evidence. *Prev Med* **20**: 47–63 (reprinted *Int J Epidemiol* **33**: 445–453).
Stampfer MJ, Hennekens CH, Manson JE, Colditz GA, Rosner B, Willett WC (1993). Vitamin E consumption and the risk of coronary disease in women *New Engl J Med* **328**: 1444–1449.
Vandenbroucke JP (2004). Commentary: the HRT story: vindication of old epidemiological theory. *Int J Epidemiol* **33**: 456–457.
Youngman LD, Keavney BD, Palmer A (2000). Plasma fibrinogen and fibrinogen genotypes in 4685 cases of myocardial infarction and in 6002 controls: test of causality by 'Mendelian randomization'. *Circulation* **102**(Suppl II): 31–32.

Infant Feeding and Later Obesity Risk

Berthold Koletzko, Rüdiger von Kries, Ricardo Closa Monasterolo, Joaquín Escribano Subías, Silvia Scaglioni, Marcello Giovannini, Jeannette Beyer, Hans Demmelmair, Brigitte Anton, Dariusz Gruszfeld, Anna Dobrzanska, Anne Sengier, Jean-Paul Langhendries, Marie-Françoise Rolland Cachera, and Veit Grote, for the European Childhood Obesity Trial Study Group[†]

Abstract Some 30 years ago, Günter Dörner proposed that exposure to hormones, metabolites and neurotransmitters during limited, sensitive periods of early development exert programming effects on disease risk in human adults. Early programming of long term health has since received broad scientific support and attention. For

---

B. Koletzko(✉), J. Beyer, H. Demmelmair, and B. Anton
Dr. von Hauner Children's Hospital, Ludwig-Maximilians-University of Munich, Germany
office.koletzko@med.uni-muenchen.de

R. von Kries and V. Grote
Institute of Social Paediatrics and Adolescent Medicine,
Ludwig-Maximilians-University of Munich, Germany

R.C. Monasterolo and J.E. Sabias
Universitad Rovira i Virgili, Reus, Spain

S. Scaglioni and M. Giovannini
Deptartment of Paediatrics, University of Milano, Italy

D. Gruszfeld and A. Dobrzanska
Childrens Memorial Health Institute, Warsaw, Poland

A. Sengier
Deptartment of Paediatrics, Université Libre de Bruxelles, Brussels, Belgium

J.P. Langhendries
CHC St. Vincent, Liège-Rocourt, Belgium

M.-F.R. Cachera
INSERM, U557, Bobigny, France

[†]**The European Childhood Obesity Trial Study Group:** Annick Xhonneux, Jean-Noel Van Hees, Françoise Martin (CHC St Vincent, Liège-Rocourt, Belgium); Anna Stolarczyk, Jerzy Socha, Piotr Socha, Roman Janas, Ewa Pietraszek (Children's Memorial Health Institute, Warsaw, Poland); Sabine Verwied-Jorky, Sonia Schiess, Ingrid Pawellek, Uschi Handel, Iris Hannibal, Michaela Fritsch (Dr. von Hauner Childrens Hospital, Ludwig Maximilians University of Munich, Germany); Helfried Groebe, Anna Reith, Renate Hofmann (Klinikum Nurnberg Sued, Nurnberg, Germany); Joana Hoyos, Philippe Goyens, Clotilde Carlier, Elena Dain (Université Libre de Bruxelles, Bruxelles, Belgium); Verónica Luque Moreno, Georgina Méndez Riera (Universitat Rovira i Virgili, Spain); Sabrina Tedeschi, Carlo Agostoni, Fiammetta Vecchi, Elvira Verduci (University of Milan, Italy).

B. Koletzko et al. (eds.), *Early Nutrition Programming and Health Outcomes in Later Life: Obesity and Beyond*,

example, evidence increases for programming effects of infant feeding choices on later obesity risk. Meta-analyses of observational studies indicate that breast feeding reduces the odds ratio for obesity at school age by about 20%, relative to formula feeding, even after adjustment for biological and sociodemographic confounding variables. We hypothesized that breast feeding protects against later obesity by reducing the likelihood of high weight gain in infancy, and that this protection is caused at least partly by the lower protein supply with breast milk relative to standard infant formulae (the "Early Protein Hypothesis"). These hypotheses are tested in the European Childhood Obesity Project, a randomized double blind intervention trial in more than 1,000 infants in five European countries (Belgium, Germany, Italy, Poland, Spain). Formula fed infants were randomized to receive during the first year of life infant formulae and follow-on-formulae with higher or lower protein contents. Follow-up at 2 years of age shows that lower protein supply with formula normalizes early growth relative to a breast fed reference group and to the WHO growth reference. These results demonstrate that modification of infant feeding practice has an important potential for long-term health promotion and should prompt a review of the recommendations and policies for infant formula composition.

Keywords Infant protein requirements • infant growth • insulin • insulin like growth factor I (IGF1) • metabolic programming • randomized clinical trial

Abbreviations BMI: body mass index; IGF1: insulin like growth factor 1; ROC: receiver operating curves; YI: Youden Index

1 Introduction

Evidence accumulates that metabolic events during critical time windows of pre- and postnatal development have marked modulating effects on health in later life, a concept often referred to as *programming* or *metabolic programming* (Koletzko et al. 2005a). The term *programming* was first used in this context in the scientific literature by Professor Günter Dörner, former head of the Institute of Experimental Endocrinology at the Charité Hospital, Humboldt University at Berlin, Germany, more than 30 years ago (Koletzko 2005). He concluded that the concentrations of hormones, metabolites and neurotransmitters during limited, sensitive periods of early development can pre-programme brain development and functional disorders in human adults, as well reproduction and metabolism (Dörner 1975). At that time Dörner also proposed an interaction between the genetics and environment during early development in determining later health outcomes in adulthood, a concept that only recently has been confirmed by experimental data (Koletzko et al. 2005; Schmidt et al. 2000; Ozanne et al. 2004; Plagemann 2004). This concept of early developmental plasticity has gained wide popularity following epidemiological studies documenting relationships between early markers of growth and the later risks of hypertension, diabetes and coronary heart disease in adulthood (Barker et al. 1989; Singhal and Lucas 2004; Cole 2004; Tu et al. 2005). Growth patterns in the first year of life are receiving increased attention since rapid weight gain in infancy has been associated with adverse later health outcomes (Koletzko et al. 2005; Metcalfe and Monaghan 2001), such as higher blood pressure (Bansal et al. 2008), higher rates of overweight and body fat deposition (Toschke et al. 2004; Wells 2007; Stettler 2007; Singhal and Lanigan 2007) and higher rates of diabetes (Dunger et al. 2007).

Since infant growth patterns can be modified by infant feeding practices, prospective controlled intervention trials are needed the explore the preventive potential of optimizing early nutrition for long term health, well-being and performance. If successful, such preventive interventions could markedly enhance the possible improvement of quality of life of populations, and also have a large economic benefit for societies. Therefore, major investments in research are justified to explore the effects of interventions on relevant outcomes, the effect sizes that can be achieved, and the underlying mechanisms of such early nutritional programming. A randomized controlled trial is currently being performed as part of the European Early Nutrition Programming project (www.metabolic-programming.org), to explore the effects of modified infant formula composition on the rate of early weight gain and later obesity risk.

2 Infant Feeding and Programming of Later Obesity Risk

Childhood obesity is considered a global epidemic in view of the alarming increase in its prevalence and severity, not only in affluent but also in less privileged childhood populations worldwide (Koletzko et al. 2002a, 2004; Fisberg et al. 2004). Childhood obesity has very serious short and long term consequences on quality of life, performance achieved, as well as long-term health and life expectancy. The obesity epidemic is expected to create huge costs for society due to both loss of productivity and to ensuing costs for health care and social security systems. Therefore, effective therapeutic intervention in obese children is needed, but results of available treatment concepts are less than satisfactory, and costs tend to be high (Koletzko 2004). A Cochrane review on interventions for treating obesity in children found that no conclusions on the effects of treatment strategies and their components can be drawn with confidence (Summerbell et al. 2004). Therefore, more emphasis must be put on the development, evaluation and implementation of effective primary prevention of obesity, where optimized infant feeding may be one important element that offers opportunities for contributing to prevention of later obesity risk (Koletzko et al. 2005).

2.1 Early Growth and Later Obesity Risk

McCance and Widdowson showed in the 1950s that alteration of early growth in animals by manipulation of food intake during sensitive periods of early development predetermined the animals' ultimate weight in adulthood (Ashwell 1993). In humans high birth weight has been proposed as a risk factor for later overweight (Binkin et al. 1988; Eriksson et al. 2003), which could reflect both the roles of genetics and of early priming by the intrauterine environment. Additionally, recent studies pointed to further priming of childhood overweight in the first 2 years of life by a high postnatal weight gain (Ong et al. 2000; Stettler et al. 2002, 2003, 2005; Chomtho et al. 2008).

We evaluated growth measures of some 4,235 German children aged 5 to 6 years who participated in the obligatory school entry health examination in the state of Bavaria, and for whom data on early weight, length, BMI and Ponderal Index evaluation were available based on measurements obtained at birth, 6, 12 and 24 months as part of the preventive health care checks offered to all children free of charge (Toschke et al. 2004). Overweight at school entry was assessed according to sex- and age-specific BMI cut-points. Growth measures in early life were analysed as possible predictors of later overweight by receiver operating curves (ROC) and predictive values. For all parameters the highest areas under ROC were observed for the gain between birth and 24 months. The area under ROC decreased in the order from weight gain (0.76) to BMI gain (0.69) to length gain (0.58) ($p < 0.001$) (Table 1). Thus, high weight gain during the first 24 months is the best overall predictor of overweight at school entry compared to other anthropometric markers and time intervals.

Similar to our findings, numerous studies in other populations also found rapid weight gain during infancy or the first 2 years of life associated with an increased

Table 1 Area under receiver operating characteristic (ROC) curves and cutpoints, sensitivity and specificity at highest Youden index for early anthropometric measurement prediction of overweight at school age in 4,235 children in Bavaria, Germany. Weight gain from birth to age 2 years is the best predictor of overweight at school age (Adapted from Toschke et al. 2004)

Measure	Area under ROC	Cutpoint at highest Youden index (YI)†	Sensitivity at highest YI	Specificity at highest YI
Age 0–6 months				
Weight	0.63 (0.60–0.66)	5,100 g (19)	45 (40–50)	74 (73–76)
Length	0.51 (0.48–0.55)	20 cm (4)	21 (17–25)	83 (81–84)
BMI‡	0.60 (0.57–0.63)	5 (15)	43 (38–48)	72 (70–73)
Ponderal index§	0.59 (0.53–0.60)	0.2 (11)	32 (27–37)	78 (76–79)
Age 0–12 months				
Weight	0.68 (0.65–0.70)	6,933 g (27)	68 (63–72)	59 (58–61)
Length	0.55 (0.52–0.58)	26 cm (9)	66 (61–71)	43 (42–45)
BMI‡	0.63 (0.60–0.66)	4 (20)	66 (62–71)	53 (51–55)
Ponderal index§	0.57 (0.54–0.60)	−0.3 (11)	64 (59–69)	47 (45–48)
Age 0–24 months				
Weight	0.76 (0.74–0.79)	9,764 g (41)	70 (65–75)	71 (69–72)
Length	0.58 (0.55–0.61)	39 cm (13)	45 (40–50)	68 (66–69)
BMI‡	0.70 (0.67–0.72)	4 (31)	57 (52–62)	74 (73–75)
Ponderal index§	0.61 (0.58–0.64)	−0.5 (17)	44 (39–49)	72 (71–74)

Data are given as value (95% confidence interval) unless otherwise indicated.
†(Sensitivity + specificity) − 1.
‡Calculated as weight in kilograms divided by the square of height in meters.
§Calculated as weight in kilograms divided by the length in meters cubed.

risk of later obesity. Three recent systematic reviews on the available evidence from the large number of observational studies confirmed that rapid weight gain in infancy and the first 2 years of life is a significant risk indicator for later adiposity (Baird et al. 2005; Monteiro and Victora 2005; Ong and Loos 2006). Thus, early infancy may provide an opportunity for interventions aiming at reducing later obesity risk.

3 Protective Effects of Breast Feeding Against Later Obesity

Populations of infants fed breast milk or formula show slightly different growth, with formula fed infants showing higher body weight at the end of the first year of life (Kramer et al. 2004). Based on a systematic review of 19 studies in affluent populations, Dewey concluded that the cumulative difference in body weight amounts to approximately 400 g less weight by the age of 12 months in infants breast-fed for 9 months, and as much as 600–650 g less weight at 1 year in infants that are breast-fed for 12 months (Dewey 1998). In view of this large effect of the mode of feeding on early weight gain, we aimed at studying whether breast feeding might also confer protection against later obesity risk.

In a cross sectional survey in Bavaria, Germany, we assessed the impact of breast feeding on the risk of obesity and the risk of being overweight in children at the time of entry to school (von Kries et al. 1999). Data collected on height and weight of 134,577 children participating in the obligatory health examination at the time of school entry in Bavaria were used to calculate body mass index (BMI) values, and the 90th and the 97th centile values of German children aged 5 and 6 years were calculated and served as the cutoffs to define overweight and obesity, respectively. In a subsample of 13,345 children, early feeding, diet, and lifestyle factors were assessed using responses to a questionnaire completed by parents, and data of 9,357 children aged 5 and 6 who had German nationality were included in the final analysis. Children who were never breast fed had a higher prevalence of both overweight (12.6% vs. 9.2%) and of obesity (4.5% vs. 2.8%) than children who had been breast fed. Longer duration of breast feeding was associated with a lower prevalence of later obesity: obesity prevalence was 3.8% for 2 months of breast feeding, 2.3% for 3–5 months, 1.7% for 6–12 months, and 0.8% for more than 12 months. Similar relations were found with the prevalence of being overweight. The protective effect of breast feeding was not attributable to differences in social class or lifestyle, but remained significant after adjusting for confounding factors. Compared to children who were never breastfed, those who had ever been breastfed showed a significantly reduced adjusted odds ratio for overweight (0.79, 95% confidence interval 0.68–0.93) and obesity (0.75 [0.57–0.98]). We also found an inverse dose–response relationship between duration of breastfeeding and prevalence of overweight and obesity (Fig. 1), which is compatible with a causal effect of breast feeding or breast milk components on obesity reduction.

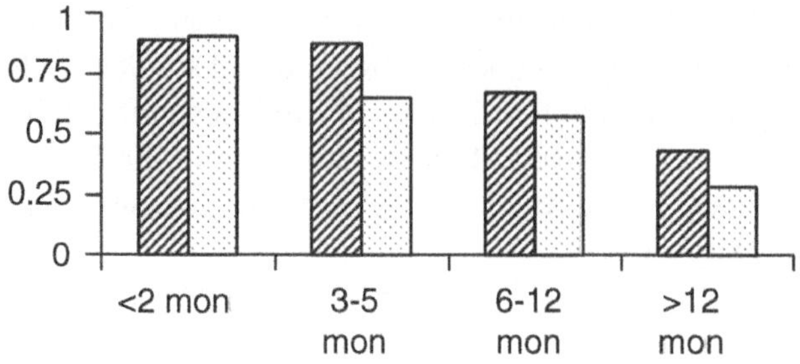

Fig. 1 Duration of breast-feeding in infancy (months) is inversely related to the odds ratio (adjusted for confounding factors) for overweight (striped bars) and obesity (light bars) at school entry in 9,357 German children (Adapted from von Kries et al. 1999)

Following our publication, many other investigators around the world evaluated the relation between breast feeding and later obesity in data collected from various cohort studies around the world. This allowed us to perform a systematic review and meta-analysis of published epidemiological studies (cohort, case-control or cross-sectional studies) evaluating effects of early feeding-mode on later overweight and obesity (Arenz et al. 2004). We limited studies to those who adjusted for at least three of the relevant confounding or interacting factors birth weight, parental overweight, parental smoking, dietary factors, physical activity and socioeconomic status. We accepted parental education as an appropriate indicator of socioeconomic status. Other inclusion criteria were: comparable risk estimates as OR or relative risk had to be reported and age at the last follow-up had to be between 5 and 18 years; feeding-mode had to be assessed and reported and obesity as outcome had to be defined by body mass index (BMI) percentiles 90, 95 or 97 to allow for comparison of the studies. We did not require all studies to use identical reference values. If risk estimates were calculated for different percentile values in a particular study, the estimate for the highest percentile-value was included in the meta-analysis. Electronic databases were searched and reference lists of relevant articles were checked. Calculations of pooled estimates were conducted in fixed-effects and random-effects models. Heterogeneity was tested by Q-test. Publication bias was assessed from funnel plots and by a linear regression method. Nine studies with more than 69,000 participants met the inclusion criteria. The meta-analysis showed that breast-feeding reduced the risk of obesity in childhood significantly. The adjusted odds ratio was 0.78 (95% CI [0.71, 0.85]) in the fixed-effects model (Fig. 2). The assumption of homogeneity of results of the included studies could not be refuted (Q-test for heterogeneity, $p > 0.3$), stratified analyses showed no differences regarding different study types, age groups, definition of breast-feeding or obesity, and number of confounding factors adjusted for. A dose dependent effect of breast-feeding duration on the prevalence of obesity was reported in four studies. Funnel plot regression gave no indication of publication bias.

Similar results were obtained by Harder and coworkers a year later in a meta-analysis with different inclusion criteria and a much larger number of evaluated studies (Harder et al. 2005). They concluded that ever breastfeeding leads to significantly reduced pooled adjusted odds ratio for later obesity of 0.75 (95% CI: 0.68–0.82), and again they found a clear dose–response effect, with each

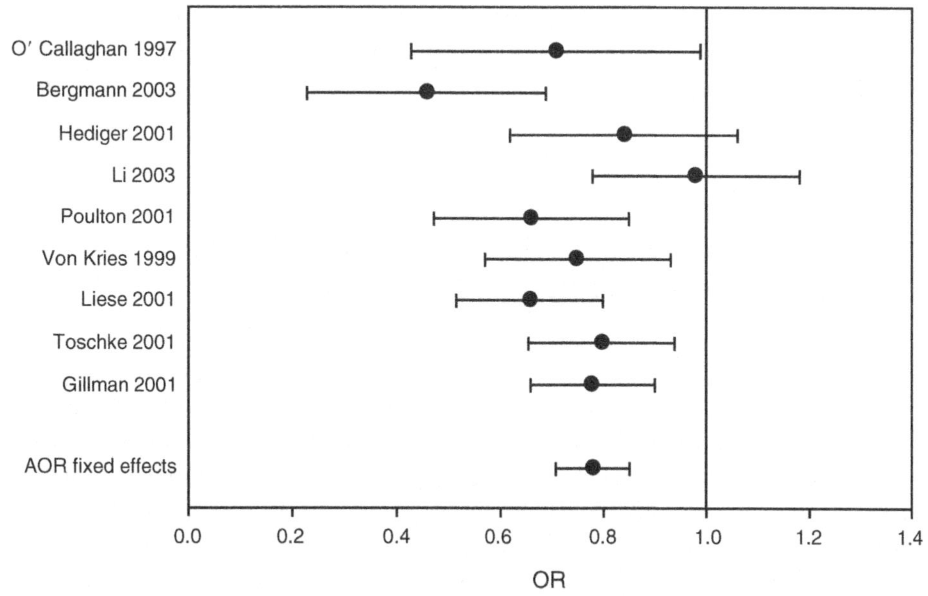

Fig. 2 Forrest plot of meta-analysis of effects of breast feeding versus formula feeding on childhood obesity: covariate-adjusted odds ratios of nine studies and pooled adjusted odds ratio (Adapted from Arenz et al. 2004)

additional month of breast feeding reducing later obesity risk by a further 4%. A further meta-analysis published thereafter also confirmed a protective effect of breast feeding, but reported a smaller effect size with an odds ratio of 0.87 (Owen et al. 2005). This result was primarily due to the data of one publication based on the population of the Women, Infants and Children program in the USA (WIC) supporting low-income women and children, which contributed 75% of the total weight of all studies, and the question has been raised whether specific aspects in this cohort such as a high degree of mixed feeding might explain these results. One cluster randomized study performed in Belarus had randomized hospitals to a program of breast feeding intervention or no active intervention, and it achieved a significantly longer duration of breastfeeding with the intervention (Kramer et al. 2007). When the children were revisited at the age of 6.5 years, measures of obesity in the intervention and control groups were not significantly different. However, in this study basically all children had been breastfed, and while the intervention modified the duration of breastfeeding the study does not allow conclusions on the effect of breast versus formula feeding. Moreover, the prevalence of obesity was rather low in this population, and the overall power of the study to detect effects on obesity is not high.

The consistent finding of a modest but significant protective effect of breastfeeding on later obesity in numerous observational studies and in three meta-analysis is encouraging and may contribute to promoting, protection and support of breastfeeding. However, it appears worthwhile to elucidate the potential underlying mechanisms for protection by breastfeeding because this would strengthen the conclusions on apparent protective effects, and it might help to extend protective effects to populations of infants that are not benefiting from long duration of full breastfeeding.

4 Potential Causative Mechanisms for the Protective Effects of Breast Feeding on Later Obesity

A number of hypotheses could be raised with respect to potential causes for a protective effect of breast feeding on later obesity risk. Even though the inverse relationship of both breast feeding and breast feeding duration with later obesity was shown to persist in many studies after adjustment for measurable confounding variables, residual confounding cannot be fully excluded. Since healthy babies can generally not be randomised to breastfeeding or formula feeding for ethical and practical reasons, undisputable proof for a causal protective effect of breastfeeding is difficult to obtain. However, the consistent results of many studies and the dose–response relationship between longer duration of breast feeding and greater later reduction of obesity risk observed in a number of studies make it likely that there is a causal effect of breast feeding.

4.1 Differences in Behaviour

Differences in feeding behaviour and mother–child-interaction between populations of breast and formula fed infants might play a role. Breast fed infants show a different suckling pattern and a higher suckling frequency (Mathew and Bhatia 1989; Bosma et al. 1990). Breast fed infants seem to have greater degree of control on meal sizes and intervals than infants fed formula. Sievers and coworkers monitored marked differences in feeding patterns, with a 20–30% higher feeding volume in formula fed infants after 6 weeks of life as well as a smaller number of total meals and of nightly meals in bottle fed babies at 4 months of age (Sievers et al. 2002). Such early differences in feeding behaviour might be related to later body size. Agras and coworkers reported that early feeding patterns were predictive of body mass index at 3 years of age, with high-pressure sucking measured in the laboratory at 2 and 4 weeks of age (denoting a vigorous feeding style) associated with greater degree of adiposity in toddlers (Agras et al. 1990).

In contrast to infant formula, breast milk shows marked variation in its composition, taste and smell from day to day, and even from meal to meal, depending on maternal dietary habits and other metabolic factors, as well as duration of lactation, the volume of milk consumed and the degree of breast expression (Rodriguez et al. 1999). Since early taste experience in infancy has been reported to favour later consumption of foods with the same taste (Mennella et al. 2001), it is conceivable that breast fed infants might be programmed to different food selection and dietary habits in alter life.

Breastfeeding is believed to enhance emotional bonding of the mother to her child, mediated in part by the stimulation of maternal oxytocin release by infant suckling, and breastfeeding mothers have decreased neuroendocrine response to stressors, increased parasympathetic nervous system modulation, lower perceived stress levels and fewer depressive symptoms (Klaus, 1998; Mezzacappa, 2004). These effects of breast feeding might well have repercussions on the interaction between mother and child and health related behaviours. These and further behavioural hypotheses are plausible and attractive, and they deserve further exploration, even though experimental testing of these hypotheses may not be easy.

4.2 Differences in Milk Composition

While the mode of feeding an infant at the breast cannot be copied with bottle feeding of human milk substitutes, some of the compositional differences and substrate supply between breastmilk and infant formula might potentially be reduced by appropriate modifications of infant formula composition. Promising hypotheses can be deduced from studies evaluating physiological responses of breast and bottle fed infants. We hypothesized that the higher rates of weight gain in populations of formula fed infants, as compared to infants fed human milk, are at least partly due to differences in metabolizable protein intakes (Koletzko et al. 2005).

Infant formulae tend to have a higher average caloric density (kcal/100 ml) than average values for breast milk, and energy supplies per kg bodyweight between 3 and 12 months of age are 10–18% higher in formula fed infants than in breastfed babies (Heinig et al. 1993). However, much greater is the difference in protein intake per kg bodyweight, which is 55–80% higher in formula than in breast fed infants (Fig. 3) (Alexy et al. 1999). In rats, prenatal high protein exposure decreased energy expenditure and increased later adiposity (Daenzer et al. 2002), and a high postnatal protein and nutrient supply led to higher adult body fat deposition (Kim et al. 1991) and increased adult weight by 10–40% (Jones et al. 1984). A high protein intake in excess of metabolic requirements may enhance the secretion of insulin and insulin like growth factor 1 (IGF1) (Fig. 4). Infants fed cows' milk protein based infant formula were shown to have far higher postprandial levels of insulin on day 6 of life than breastfed infants (Lucas et al. 1981). High insulin and IGF1 values can enhance both growth during the first 2 years of life (Karlberg et al. 1994; Hoppe et al. 2004a) as well as adipogenic activity and adipocyte differentiation (Hauner et al. 1989) (Fig. 4). High protein intakes may also decrease human growth hormone (hGH) secretion and lipolysis. Some epidemiological studies showed a significant relationship of high protein intakes in early childhood, but not of the intakes of energy, fat or carbohydrates, to an early occurrence of the adiposity rebound and to a high childhood body mass index (BMI), corrected for parental BMI (Rolland-Cachera et al. 1995;

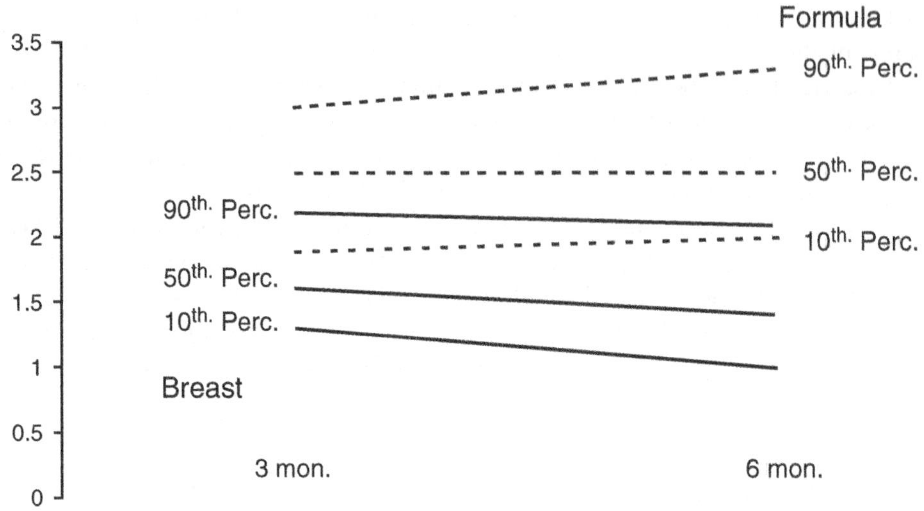

Fig. 3 Percentiles of protein intake (g/kg and day) of healthy breastfed and formula fed infants at the ages of 3 and 6 months (median and 90th/10th percentiles). Data of the German DONALD study (Redrawn from data of Alexy et al. 1999)

Parizkova and Rolland-Cachera 1997; Scaglioni et al. 2000; Hoppe et al. 2004b). These and other data support our hypothesis that a higher protein intake with infant formula than provided with breast milk and in excess of metabolic requirements may predispose to an increased obesity risk in later life (the Early Protein Hypothesis) (Koletzko et al. 2005).

5 Testing the Early Protein Hypothesis: The European Childhood Obesity Project

In addition to prospective epidemiological and experimental studies, human intervention trials are needed to test the "Early Protein Hypothesis". The European Childhood Obesity Project (www.metabolic-programming.org) funded by the European Commission's fifth Framework Research Programme and sixth Framework Research Programme was set up to test, in a randomized double blind intervention trial, whether higher or lower protein intakes during the first year of life influence growth until the age of 2 years and obesity risk at school age. This trial is conducted in five European countries (Belgium, Germany, Italy, Poland, Spain) which differ substantially in the practice of infant and young child feeding and in their prevalence of adult obesity. Therefore the trial offers the opportunity to combine a multicentre intervention trial on infant formulae which differ in their balance of protein and fat (provided by Bledina, Steenvoorde, France), with an epidemiological observation study which can assess protein intake in the overall early diet. We anticipate that this approach will enable us to assess the effects of

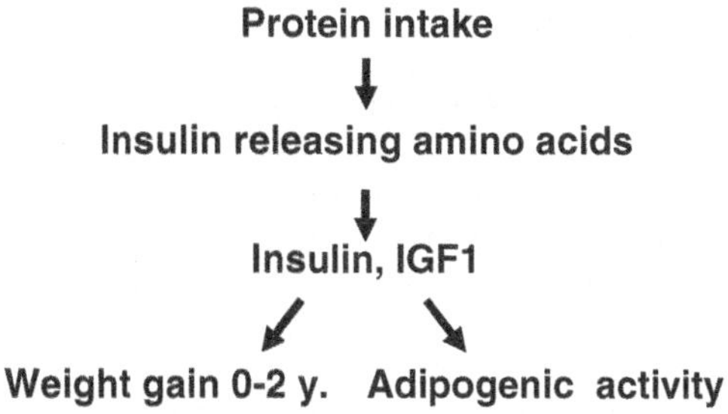

Fig. 4 High protein intakes with infant formula may induce high circulating concentrations of insulin releasing amino acids, which may stimulate the secretion of insulin and insulin like growth factor 1 and hence induce both an enhanced weight gain from birth to 2 years of life as well as enhanced adipogenic activity

variables which differ substantially within Europe, as well as to assess the effects of the randomized controlled intervention. The inclusion of a group of breastfed infants in each centre will also allow an epidemiological comparison of the effects of breastfeeding and formula feeding.

Growth from birth to age 2 years, a marker of later obesity risk, was chosen as the primary outcome variable, based on our previous findings that this is a predictive marker of later obesity risk (Toschke et al. 2004). In addition, a variety of further variables are measured, including detailed data on diet, lifestyle and behaviour, biochemical and endocrine markers, markers of renal function, and others. Randomisation and data collection are performed via the internet based on uniform electronic case report forms, using specially developed information technology architecture with a central database and 12 remote data entry stations as well as dedicated software that allows for secure data protection. Mechanisms for quality assurance have also been established. Data input and transfer to the central database are supervised by a contract research organization participating in the project.

Recruitment for the intervention and follow-up until the age of 2 years has been successfully completed. The first data evaluation indicates that the group of infants randomized to the formulas with higher protein contents show a significantly higher body weight and body mass index at the age of 2 years than the group of infants randomized to lower protein supply (Koletzko et al. submitted 2008). Provision of the lower protein content with formula led to normalized growth measures at 2 years, relative to the breast fed reference group. Further data evaluation is ongoing, and the subjects in the trial are being followed up to explore both the longer-term safety as well as the potential benefits of the intervention at preschool and school age. Based on the available data from observational trials, we expect that the reduction of weight for length achieved at 2 years with the lower protein supply may reduce later obesity risk by some 10–15%. However, even the early results obtained might lead to a review of recommendations for infant feeding, policy and regulatory guidance, as well as product design, since the aim is for physiological growth of formula fed populations similar to the growth of healthy breastfed populations (Koletzko et al. 2002b), and there is no known advantage of growth patterns of formula fed babies that deviate from the model of breastfed populations.

Acknowledgments The authors thank the participating families and all project partners for their enthusiastic support of the project work, and Wm. Cameron Chumlea, Ph.D., Fels Professor, Departments of Community Health and Pediatrics, Lifespan Health Research Center, Wright State University Boonshoft School of Medicine, Dayton, OH, for his help in setting up standardized anthropometric measures and in training the study personnel. The studies reported herein have been carried out with partial financial support from the Commission of the European Communities, specific RTD Programme "Quality of Life and Management of Living Resources", within the 5th Framework Programme, research grants no. QLRT-2001-00389 and QLK1-CT-2002-30582, and the 6th Framework Programme, contract no. 007036. This manuscript does not necessarily reflect the views of the Commission and in no way anticipates the future policy in this area. Additional support from the Child Health Foundation, Munich, the LMU innovative research priority project MC-Health (sub-project I), and the International Danone Institutes is gratefully acknowledged. BK is the recipient of a Freedom to Discover Award of the Bristol-Myers-Squibb Foundation, New York, NY, USA.

Statement on conflicts of interest

The author declares that there is no conflict of interest, following the definitions in the guidance of the International Committee of Medical Journal Editors (http://www.icmje.org/).

References

Agras WS, Kraemer HC, Berkowitz RI, Hammer LD (1990, May). Influence of early feeding style on adiposity at 6 years of age. *J Pediatr* **116**(5): 805–809.

Alexy U, Kersting M, Sichert-Hellert W, Manz F, Schöch G (1999). Macronutrient intake of 3- to 36-month-old German infants and children: results of the DONALD Study. Dortmund Nutritional and Anthropometric Longitudinally Designed Study. *Ann Nutr Metab* **43**(1): 14–22.

Arenz S, Rückerl R, Koletzko B, von Kries R (2004). Breast-feeding and childhood obesity. A systematic review. *Int J Obes* **28**: 1247–1256.

Ashwell M (ed.). McCance & Widdowson (1993). *A scientific partnership for 60 years*. London: The British Nutrition Foundation.

Baird J, Fisher D, Lucas P, Kleijnen J, Roberts H, Law C (2005). Being big or growing fast: systematic review of size and growth in infancy and later obesity. *Brit Med J* **331**(7522): 929–931.

Bansal N, Ayoola OO, Gemmell I, Vyas A, Koudsi A, Oldroyd J, Clayton PE, Cruickshank JK (2008, Mar). Effects of early growth on blood pressure of infants of British European and South Asian origin at one year of age: the Manchester children's growth and vascular health study. *J Hypertens* **26**(3): 412–418.

Barker DJ, Osmond C, Golding J, Kuh D, Wadsworth ME (1989, Mar 4). Growth in utero, blood pressure in childhood and adult life, and mortality from cardiovascular disease. *BMJ* **298**(6673): 564–567.

Binkin NJ, Yip R, Fleshood L, Trowbridge FL (1988, Dec). Birth weight and childhood growth. *Pediatrics* **82**(6): 828–834.

Bosma JF, Hepburn LG, Josell SD, Baker K (1990, Mar). Ultrasound demonstration of tongue motions during suckle feeding. *Dev Med Child Neurol* **32**(3): 223–229.

Chomtho S, Wells JC, Williams JE, Davies PS, Lucas A, Fewtrell MS (2008, Jun). Infant growth and later body composition: evidence from the 4-component model. *Am J Clin Nutr* **87**(6): 1776–1784.

Cole TJ (2004, Jan). Modeling postnatal exposures and their interactions with birth size. *J Nutr* **134**(1): 201–204.

Daenzer M, Ortmann S, Klaus S, Metges CC (2002, Feb). Prenatal high protein exposure decreases energy expenditure and increases adiposity in young rats. *J Nutr* **132**(2): 142–144.

Dewey KG (1998). Growth characteristics of breast-fed compared to formula-fed infants. *Biol Neonate* **74**(2): 94–105.

Dörner G (1975). Perinatal hormone levels and brain organization. In: Stumpf WE, Grant LD (eds.), *Anatomical neuroendocrinology*. Basel: Karger, pp. 245–252.

Dunger DB, Salgin B, Ong KK (2007, Aug). Session 7: early nutrition and later health early developmental pathways of obesity and diabetes risk. *Proc Nutr Soc* **66**(3): 451–457.

Eriksson J, Forsen T, Osmond C, Barker D (2003, Jun). Obesity from cradle to grave. *Int J Obes Relat Metab Disord* **27**(6): 722–727.

Fisberg M, Baur L, Chen W, Nelson T, Koletzko B, Moreno L, Uauy R, Hoppin R, Lau D, Strauss R (2004). Childhood obesity – a global perspective. *J Pediatr Gastro Nutr* **39**: S678–S687.

Harder T, Bergmann R, Kallischnigg G, Plagemann A (2005, Sep 1). Duration of breastfeeding and risk of overweight: a meta-analysis. *Am J Epidemiol* **162**(5): 397–403.

Hauner H, Wabitsch M, Zwiauer K, Widhalm K, Pfeiffer EF (1989). Adipogenic activity in sera from obese children before and after weight reduction. *Am J Clin Nutr* **50**(1): 63–67.

Heinig MJ, Nommsen LA, Peerson JM, Lonnerdal B, Dewey KG (1993, Aug). Energy and protein intakes of breast-fed and formula-fed infants during the first year of life and their association with growth velocity: the DARLING Study. *Am J Clin Nutr* **58**(2): 152–161.

Hoppe C, Udam TR, Lauritzen L, Molgaard C, Juul A, Michaelsen KF (2004a, Aug). Animal protein intake, serum insulin-like growth factor I, and growth in healthy 2.5-y-old Danish children. *Am J Clin Nutr* **80**(2): 447–452.

Hoppe C, Molgaard C, Thomsen BL, Juul A, Michaelsen KF (2004b, Mar). Protein intake at 9 mo of age is associated with body size but not with body fat in 10-y-old Danish children. *Am J Clin Nutr* **79**(3): 494–501.

Jones A, Simson E, Friedman M (1984). Gestational undernutrition and the development of obesity in rats. *J Nutr* **114**: 1484–1492.

Karlberg J, Jalil F, Lam B, Low L, Yeung CY (1994). Linear growth retardation in relation to the three phases of growth. *Eur J Clin Nutr* **48**(Suppl 1): S25–S43.

Kim S, Mauron J, Gleason R, Wurtman R (1991). Selection of carbohydrate to protein ratio and correlations with weight gain and body fat in rats allowed three dietary choices. *Int J Vit Nutr Res* **61**: 166–179.

Klaus M (1998, Nov). Mother and infant: early emotional ties. *Pediatrics* **102**(5 Suppl E): 1244–1246.

Koletzko B (2004). Childhood obesity: time for treatment or prevention? *Eur J Lipid Sci Technol* **106**: 287–288.

Koletzko B (2005). Developmental origins of adult disease: Barker's or Dörner's hypothesis? *Am J Hum Biol* **17**: 381–382.

Koletzko B, Girardet JP, Klish W, Tabacco O (2002a). Obesity in children and adolescents worldwide: current views and future directions. *J Pediatr Gastroenterol Nutr* **35**: S205–S212.

Koletzko B, Ashwell M, Beck B, Bronner A, Mathioudakis B (2002b). Characterisation of infant food modifications in the European Union. *Ann Nutr Metab* **46**: 231–242.

Koletzko B, de la Guéronnière V, Toschke AM, von Kries R (2004). Nutrition in children and adolescents in Europe: what is the scientific basis? Introduction. *Brit J Nutr* **92**(Suppl 2):S67–S73.

Koletzko B, Akerblom H, Dodds PF, Ashwell M (Hrsg.) (2005a) Early nutrition and its later consequences: new opportunities. New York, Springer. *Adv Exp Med Biol* **569**: 1–237.

Koletzko B, Broekaert I, Demmelmair H, Franke J, Hannibal I, Oberle D, Schiess S, Troy Baumann B, Verwied-Jorky S (2005b). Protein intake in the first year of life: a risk factor for later obesity? In: Koletzko B, Akerblom H, Dodds PF, Ashwell M (Hrsg.), *Early nutrition and its later consequences: new opportunities. Adv Exp Med Biol* **569**: 70–79.

Kramer MS, Guo T, Platt RW, Vanilovich I, Sevkovskaya Z, Dzikovich I, Michaelsen KF, Dewey K (2004, Nov). Promotion of Breastfeeding Intervention Trials Study Group. Feeding effects on growth during infancy. *J Pediatr* **145**(5): 600–605.

Kramer MS, Matush L, Vanilovich I, Platt RW, Bogdanovich N, Sevkovskaya Z, Dzikovich I, Shishko G, Collet JP, Martin RM, Davey Smith G, Gillman MW, Chalmers B, Hodnett E, Shapiro S, PROBIT Study Group (2007, Dec). Effects of prolonged and exclusive breastfeeding on child height, weight, adiposity, and blood pressure at age 6.5 y: evidence from a large randomized trial. *Am J Clin Nutr* **86**(6): 1717–1721.

Lucas A, Boyes S, Bloom SR, Aynsley-Green A (1981, Mar). Metabolic and endocrine responses to a milk feed in six-day-old term infants: differences between breast and cow's milk formula feeding. *Acta Paediatr Scand* **70**(2): 195–200.

Mathew OP, Bhatia J (1989, May). Sucking and breathing patterns during breast- and bottle-feeding in term neonates. Effects of nutrient delivery and composition. *Am J Dis Child* **143**(5): 588–592.

Mennella JA, Jagnow CP, Beauchamp GK (2001, Jun). Prenatal and postnatal flavor learning by human infants. *Pediatrics* **107**(6): E88.

Metcalfe NB, Monaghan P (2001). Compensation for a bad start: grow now, pay later? *Trends Ecol Evol* **16**(5): 254–260.

Mezzacappa ES (2004, Jul). Breastfeeding and maternal stress response and health. *Nutr Rev* **62**(7 Pt 1): 261–268.

Monteiro POA, Victora CG (2005). Rapid growth in infancy and childhood and obesity in later life – a systematic review. *Obes Rev* **6**(2): 143–154.

Ong KK, Loos RJF (2006). Rapid infancy weight gain and subsequent obesity: systematic reviews and hopeful suggestions. *Acta Paediatr* **95**(8): 904–908.

Ong KK, Ahmed ML, Emmett PM, Preece MA, Dunger DB (2000, Apr 8). Association between postnatal catch-up growth and obesity in childhood: prospective cohort study. *BMJ* **320**(7240): 967–971.

Owen CG, Martin RM, Whincup PH, Smith GD, Cook DG (2005, May). Effect of infant feeding on the risk of obesity across the life course: a quantitative review of published evidence. *Pediatrics* **115**(5): 1367–1377.

Ozanne SE, Fernandez-Twinn D, Hales CN (2004, Feb). Fetal growth and adult diseases. *Semin Perinatol* **28**(1): 81–87.

Parizkova J, Rolland-Cachera M (1997). High proteins early in life as a predisposition for later obesity and further health risks. *Nutrition* **13**: 818–819.

Plagemann A (2004). 'Fetal programming'and 'functional teratogenesis': on epigenetic mechanisms and prevention of perinatally acquired lasting health risks. *J Perinat Med* **32**: 297–305.

Rodriguez M, Koletzko B, Kunz C, Jensen R (1999). Nutritional and biochemical properties of human milk, part II. Lipids, micronutrients and bioactive factors. *Clin Perinatol* **26**: 335–359.

Rolland-Cachera MF, Deheeger M, Akrout M, Bellisle F (1995). Influence of macronutrients on adiposity development: a follow-up study of nutrition and growth from 10 months to 8 years of age. *Int J Obes Metab Disord* **19**(8): 573–578.

Scaglioni S, Agostoni C, DeNotaris R et al. (2000) Early macronutrient intake and overweight at five years of age. *Int J Obes* **24**: 777–781.

Schmidt I, Schoelch C, Ziska T, Schneider D, Simon E, Plagemann A (2000). Interaction of genetic and environmental programming of the leptin system and of obesity disposition. *Am J Physiol Physiol Genom* **3**: 113–120.

Sievers E, Oldigs HD, Santer R, Schaub J (2002). Feeding patterns in breast-fed and formula-fed infants. *Ann Nutr Metab* **46**(6): 243–248.

Singhal A, Lanigan J (2007). Breastfeeding, early growth and later obesity. *Obes Rev* **8**: 51–54.

Singhal A, Lucas A (2004, May 15). Early origins of cardiovascular disease: is there a unifying hypothesis? *Lancet* **363**(9421): 1642–1645.

Stettler N (2007, Jul). Nature and strength of epidemiological evidence for origins of childhood and adulthood obesity in the first year of life. *Int J Obes (Lond)* **31**(7): 1035–1043.

Stettler N, Zemel BS, Kumanyika S, Stallings VA (2002, Feb). Infant weight gain and childhood overweight status in a multicenter, cohort study. *Pediatrics* **109**(2): 194–199.

Stettler N, Kumanyika SK, Katz SH, Zemel BS, Stallings VA (2003, Jun). Rapid weight gain during infancy and obesity in young adulthood in a cohort of African Americans. *Am J Clin Nutr* **77**(6): 1374–1378.

Stettler N, Stallings VA, Troxel AB, Zhao J, Schinnar R, Nelson SE, Ziegler EE, Strom BL (2005, Apr 19). Weight gain in the first week of life and overweight in adulthood: a cohort study of European American subjects fed infant formula. *Circulation* **111**(15): 1897–1903.

Summerbell CD, Ashton V, Campbell KJ, Edmunds L, Kelly S, Waters E (2003). Interventions for treating obesity in children. Cochrane Database Syst Rev. 2003(3): CD001872. PMID: 12917914.

Toschke AM, Grote V, Koletzko B, von Kries R (2004, May). Identifying children at high risk for overweight at school entry by weight gain during the first 2 years. *Arch Pediatr Adolesc Med* **158**(5): 449–452.

Tu YK, West R, Ellison GT, Gilthorpe MS (2005, Jan 1). Why evidence for the fetal origins of adult disease might be a statistical artifact: the "reversal paradox" for the relation between birth weight and blood pressure in later life. *Am J Epidemiol* **161**(1): 27–32.

von Kries R, Koletzko B, Sauerwald T, von Mutius E, Barnert D, Grunert V, von Voss H (1999). Breastfeeding and obesity: cross sectional study. *Brit Med J* **319**: 147–150.

Wells JC (2007, Dec). The programming effects of early growth. *Early Hum Dev* **83**(12): 743–748. Epub 2007 Sep 29.

Developmental Origins of Osteoporosis: The Role of Maternal Nutrition

Cyrus Cooper, Nicholas Harvey, Zoe Cole, Mark Hanson, and Elaine Dennison

Abstract Osteoporosis is a major cause of morbidity and mortality through its association with age-related fractures. Although most effort in fracture prevention has been directed at retarding the rate of age-related bone loss, and reducing the frequency and severity of trauma among elderly people, evidence is growing that peak bone mass is an important contributor to bone strength during later life. The normal patterns of skeletal growth have been well characterised in cross-sectional and longitudinal studies. It has been confirmed that boys have higher bone mineral content, but not volumetric bone density, than girls. Furthermore, there is a dissociation between the peak velocities for height gain and bone mineral accrual in both genders. Puberty is the period during which volumetric density appears to increase in both axial and appendicular sites. Many factors influence the accumulation of bone mineral during childhood and adolescence, including heredity, gender, diet, physical activity, endocrine status, and sporadic risk factors such as cigarette smoking. In addition to these modifiable factors during childhood, evidence has also accrued that fracture risk might be programmed during intrauterine life. Epidemiological studies have demonstrated a relationship between birthweight, weight in infancy, and adult bone mass. This appears to be mediated through modulation of the set-point for basal activity of pituitary-dependent endocrine systems such as the hypothalamic-pituitary-adrenal (HPA) and growth hormone/insulin-like growth factor-1 (GH/IGF-1) axes. Maternal smoking, diet (particularly vitamin D deficiency) and physical activity also appear to modulate bone mineral acquisition during intrauterine life; furthermore, both low birth size and poor childhood growth, are directly linked to the later risk of hip fracture. The optimisation of maternal nutrition and intrauterine growth should also be included within preventive strategies against osteoporotic fracture, albeit for future generations.

C. Cooper(✉), N. Harvey, Z. Cole, M. Hanson, and E. Dennison
MRC Epidemiology Resource Centre and Centre for Developmental Origins of Health and Adult Disease, University of Southampton, Southampton General Hospital, Southampton SO16 6YD
cc@mrc.soton.ac.uk

B. Koletzko et al. (eds.), *Early Nutrition Programming and Health Outcomes in Later Life: Obesity and Beyond*,

Keywords Epidemiology • osteoporosis • fetal origins • bone mineral

Abbreviations BMC: bone mineral content; BMD: bone mineral density; DXA: dual-energy x-ray absorptiometry; GH: growth hormone; HPA: hypothalamic-pituitary-adrenal; IGF: insulin-like growth factor; WBBMC: whole body bone mineral content

1 Introduction

Osteoporosis is a skeletal disorder characterised by low bone mass and micro-architectural deterioration of bone tissue with a consequent increase in bone fragility and susceptibility to fracture (Consensus Development Conference 1991; Cooper 2003). The risk of osteoporotic fracture ultimately depends on two factors: the mechanical strength of bone and the forces applied to it. Bone mass (a composite measure including contributions from bone size and from its volumetric mineral density) is an established determinant of bone strength, and the bone mass of an individual in later life depends upon the peak attained during skeletal growth and the subsequent rate of bone loss. Several longitudinal studies attest to the tracking of bone mass through childhood and adolescence, and mathematical models suggest that modifying peak bone mass will have biologically relevant effects on skeletal fragility in old age. There is evidence to suggest that peak bone mass is inherited, but current genetic markers are able to explain only a small proportion of the variation in individual bone mass or fracture risk (Ralston 1998).

Environmental influences during childhood and puberty have been shown to benefit bone mineral accrual, but the relatively rapid rate of mineral gain during intrauterine and early postnatal life, coupled with the plasticity of skeletal development in utero, offer the possibility of profound interactions between the genome and early environment at this stage in the life course. There is a strong biological basis for such a model of disease pathogenesis. Experimentalists have repeatedly demonstrated that minor alterations to the diet of pregnant animals can produce lasting changes in the body build, physiology and metabolism of the offspring (Bateson 2001). This is one example of a ubiquitous phenomenon (phenotypic or developmental plasticity), which enables one genotype to give rise to a range of different physiological or morphological states in response to different prevailing environmental conditions during development. Its essence lies in the critical period during which a system is plastic and sensitive to the environment, followed by a loss of that plasticity and a fixed functional capacity. The evolutionary benefit of the phenomenon is that in a changing environment, it maximises phenotypic diversity and enables the production of phenotypes that are better matched to their environment than would be possible with the production of the same phenotype in all environments. This review will address the role played by influences during intrauterine or early postnatal life in establishing the risk of osteoporosis in later years. It will cover the epidemiological evidence linking the risk of low bone density and fracture to environmental influences during early development; the impact of maternal nutrition and lifestyle on intrauterine bone mineral accrual; and the mechanisms underlying the relationship between developmental plasticity and osteoporosis.

2 Developmental Origins of Osteoporosis

Epidemiological studies of coronary heart disease performed over a decade ago demonstrated strong geographic associations between death rate from the disorder in 1968–1978, and infant mortality in 1901–1910. Subsequent research, based on individuals whose birth records had been preserved for 7 decades, revealed that men and women who were undernourished during intrauterine life, and therefore had low birthweight or were thin at birth, had an increased risk for coronary heart disease, hypertension, non-insulin dependent diabetes, and hypercholesterolaemia (Barker 1995). These associations are explained by a phenomenon known as programming (Lucas 1991); this term describes persisting changes in structure and function caused by environmental stimuli acting at critical periods during early development. During embryonic life, the basic form of the human baby is laid down in miniature. However, the body does not increase greatly in size until the fetal period when a rapid growth phase commences, which continues until after birth. The main feature of fetal growth is cell division. Different tissues of the body grow during periods of rapid cell division, so called 'critical' periods (Widdowson and McCance 1974).

Evidence that the risk of osteoporosis might be modified by environmental influences during early life stems from four groups of studies: (a) bone mineral measurements undertaken in cohorts of adults whose detailed birth and/or childhood records have been preserved; (b) detailed physiological studies exploring the relationship between candidate endocrine systems which might be programmed (GH/IGF-1; hypothalamic-pituitary adrenal, gonadal steroid) and age-related bone loss; (c) studies characterising the nutrition, body build and lifestyle of pregnant women and relating these to the bone mass of their newborn offspring; and (d) studies relating childhood growth rates to the later risk of hip fracture.

2.1 Population Studies

The first epidemiological evidence that osteoporosis risk might be programmed came from a study of 153 women born in Bath during 1968–1969 who were traced and studied at age 21 years (Cooper et al. 1995). Data on childhood growth were obtained from linked birth and school health records. There were statistically significant ($p < 0.05$) associations between weight at 1 year and bone mineral content (BMC), but not density (BMD), at the lumbar spine and femoral neck; these relationships were independent of adult weight and body mass index. The data suggested a discordance between the processes which govern skeletal growth, and those which influence mineralization. They also provided direct evidence that the trajectory of bone growth might be modified in utero, an assertion previously only supported by inference from measurements of body height. The association between weight in infancy and adult bone mass was replicated in subsequent cohort studies of men and women aged 60–75 years, who were born and still lived in Hertfordshire (Cooper et al. 1997; Dennison et al. 2005). These studies showed highly significant relationships between weight at 1 year and adult bone area at the spine and hip ($p<0.005$); the relationships with BMC at these two sites were weaker but remained statistically significant ($p<0.02$). They also remained after adjustment for known genetic markers of osteoporosis risk, such as polymorphisms in the gene for the vitamin D receptor (Keen et al. 1997), and after adjustment for lifestyle characteristics in adulthood which might have influenced bone mass (physical activity, dietary calcium intake, cigarette smoking, and alcohol consumption).

More detailed analyses of the interactions between polymorphism in the gene for the vitamin D receptor, birthweight, and bone mineral density, have been published from the same cohort study (Dennison et al. 2001). These suggest that genetic influences on adult bone size and mineral density may be modified by undernutrition in utero. Subsequent studies from the United States, Australia and Scandinavia have replicated these relationships between weight in infancy and adult bone mass. Finally, a recent twin study (Antoniades et al. 2003) evaluated the relationship between birthweight and bone mass among 4,008 white female twins aged 47.5 years. Statistically significant relationships were found between the intra-pair differences in birthweight and in BMC, after adjustment for height and weight, even among monozygous twin pairs. These data suggest that even in genetically identical subjects, a relationship can be detected between birthweight and adult bone mass.

2.2 Physiological Studies

To explore further the potential role of hypothalamic-pituitary function and its relevance to the pathogenesis of osteoporosis, profiles of circulating GH and cortisol were compared with bone density among groups of men and women whose birth records had been preserved. These studies revealed that birthweight and weight in infancy were predictors of basal levels of GH and cortisol during late adult life (Antoniades et al. 2003; Fall et al. 1998; Dennison et al. 1999). The levels of these two skeletally active hormones were also found to be determinants of prospectively determined bone loss rate. The data are compatible with the hypothesis that environmental stressors during intrauterine or early postnatal life alter the sensitivity of the growth plate to GH and cortisol. The consequence of such endocrine programming would be to reduce peak skeletal size, perhaps also to reduce mineralization, and to predispose to an accelerated rate of bone loss during later life (Fall et al. 1998;

Dennison et al. 1999; Phillips et al. 1998). Recent studies suggest that interactions between the genome and early environment might establish basal levels of circulating GH, and thereby contribute to accelerated bone loss (Dennison et al. 2004). A single nucleotide polymorphism has been discovered at locus GH1-A5157G in the promoter region of the human growth hormone (GH1) gene. This is associated with significantly lower basal GH concentration, lower baseline BMD and accelerated bone loss (Fig. 1). As with polymorphism in the gene for the vitamin D receptor, a significant ($p = 0.02$) interaction was observed between weight at 1 year, allelic variation at this site and bone loss rate.

2.3 *Maternal Nutrition, Lifestyle and Neonatal Bone Mineral*

The third piece of epidemiological evidence that osteoporosis might arise in part through developmental maladaptation stems from investigation of a series of mothers through pregnancy; anthropometric and lifestyle maternal characteristics were related to the bone mineral of their newborn offspring (Godfrey et al. 2001). After adjusting for sex and gestational age, neonatal bone mass was strongly, positively associated with birthweight, birth length and placental weight. Other determinants included maternal and paternal birthweight, and maternal triceps skinfold thickness at 28 weeks. Maternal smoking, and maternal energy intake at 18 weeks gestation were negatively associated with neonatal BMC at both the spine and whole body.

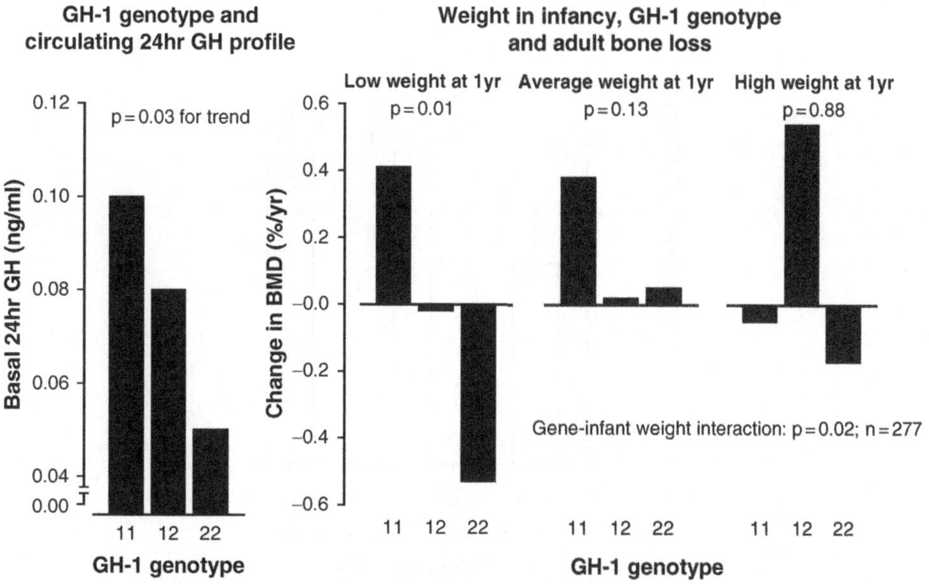

Fig. 1 GH-1 genotype, 24h GH concentration, weight in infancy and adult bone loss: Hertfordshire cohort study (Data derived from Dennison 2004)

The independent effects of maternal and paternal birthweight on fetal skeletal development support the notion that paternal influences, for example through the imprinting of growth promoting genes such as IGF-2, contribute strongly to the establishment of the early skeletal growth trajectory, while maternal nutrition and body build modify fetal nutrient supply and subsequent bone accretion, predominantly through influences on placentation.

In the most recent data from mother/offspring cohorts, body composition has been assessed by DXA in 216 children at age 9 years (Javaid et al. 2006). They and their parents had previously been included in a population-based study of maternal nutrition and fetal growth. The nutrition, body build and lifestyle of the mothers had been characterised during early and late pregnancy, and samples of umbilical venous blood had been obtained at birth. Reduced maternal height, lower pre-conceptional maternal weight, reduced maternal fat stores during late pregnancy, a history of maternal smoking and lower maternal social class were all associated with reduced whole body BMC of the child at age 9 years. Lower ionised calcium concentration in umbilical venous serum also predicted reduced childhood bone mass ($r = 0.19$, $p = 0.02$); this association appeared to mediate the effect of maternal fat stores, smoking and socio-economic status on the bone mass of the children at age 9 years. Around 25% of the mothers had sub-optimal vitamin D status as assessed by serum 25-hydroxyvitamin D concentration (Fig. 2). The children born to these mothers had significantly ($p < 0.01$) reduced whole body bone mineral content at age 9 years. This deficit in skeletal growth remained significant even after adjustment for childhood weight and bone area (Javaid et al, 2006). These data suggest that the placental capacity to maintain the materno-fetal calcium gradient

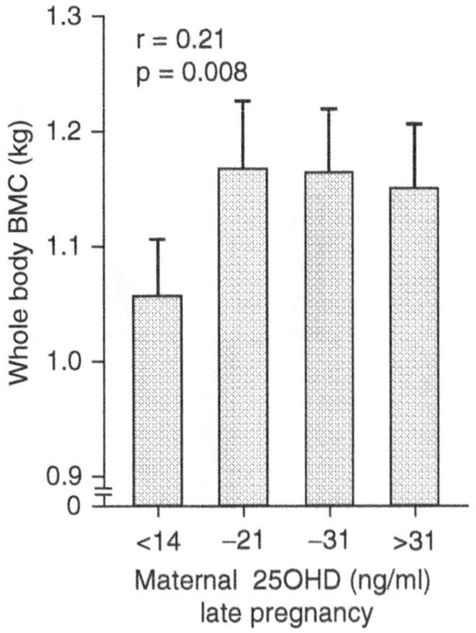

Fig. 2 Maternal 25(OHD) during late pregnancy and WBBMC of her offspring 9 years later (Data derived from Javaid et al. 2006)

is important in optimising the trajectory of postnatal skeletal growth. They are in accord with the results of follow-up studies relating vitamin D supplementation in infancy to bone mineral density in later childhood. In one such study, prepubertal Caucasian girls aged 7–9 years, who had received vitamin D supplementation during infancy, had greater areal BMD at the radius and proximal femur than a group of female controls of similar age (Zamora et al. 1999).

2.4 Childhood Growth and Hip Fracture

Most evidence relating the intrauterine environment to later osteoporosis stems from studies utilising non-invasive assessment of bone mineral. The clinically important consequence of reduced bone mass is fracture, and data are now available which directly link growth rates in childhood with the risk of later hip fracture (Cooper et al. 2001). Studies of a unique Finnish cohort in whom birth and childhood growth data were linked to later hospital discharge records for hip fracture, have permitted follow-up of around 7,000 men and women who were born in Helsinki University Central Hospital during 1924–1933. Body size at birth was recorded and an average of ten measurements were obtained of height and weight throughout childhood. Hip fracture incidence was assessed in this cohort using the Finnish hospital discharge registration system. After adjustment for age and sex, there were two major determinants of hip fracture risk: tall maternal height ($p < 0.001$), and low rate of childhood growth (height, $p = 0.006$; weight, $p = 0.01$). The effects of maternal height and childhood growth rate were statistically independent of each other, and remained after adjusting for socio-economic status. More important, hip fracture risk was also elevated ($p = 0.05$) among babies born short. These data suggest that hip fracture risk might be particularly elevated among children in whom growth of the skeletal envelope is forced ahead of the capacity to mineralise, a phenomenon which is accelerated during pubertal growth.

3 Developmental Plasticity and Osteoporosis

'Developmental plasticity' provides organisms with the ability to change structure and function in response to environmental cues; these responses usually operate during critical time windows and then become irreversible. Such plasticity permits a range of phenotypes to develop from a single genotype in response to environmental cues. In *Daphnia*, helmet formation (a defensive, morphological change) is dependent on the early environment and risk of predation. In the locust, *Locusta migratoria*, the wing shape and metabolic pathways are determined in the larval stage by pheromone signals indicating population density. In the axolotl, early environmental conditions determine whether the mature form will be purely aquatic or amphibious (West-Eberhard 2003). Developmental plasticity sets the template on which continued postnatal homeostatic and homeorhetic (maintaining a time-dependent process, e.g. growth trajectory) adaptation can occur.

There are several mechanisms by which environmental cues can influence the developmental programme. First, they can exert effects prior to implantation and affect gene expression, particularly by inducing epigenetic changes in the DNA. In the *agouti* mouse mutant, maternal dietary folate supplementation at conception alters the expression of the imprinted agouti gene by altering the capacity for methylation (Cooney et al. 2002). Non-imprinted genes can also undergo epigenetic change in response to the environment – the choice of exon usage in the glucocorticoid receptor gene is altered both by prenatal glucocorticoids and neonatal behavioural manipulation owing to changes in histone acetylation and DNA methylation in a transcriptional factor binding site (Weaver et al. 2004). These changes persist throughout life as manifested in altered hypothalamic-pituitary-adrenal (HPA) axis activity. Second, tissue differentiation may be altered. Prolonged *in vitro* culture of the rodent or ruminant embryo affects the allocation of blastocyst stem cells to inner cell mass or trophectoderm lineages (Gluckman and Hanson 2004). This influences the relative growth trajectories of the placenta and fetus, thus affecting fetal development in late gestation.

Developmental responses to environmental stimuli need not provide immediate advantages, but may alter the sensitivity of the organism to an anticipated future environment (Gluckman and Hanson 2004). Such predictive adaptive responses are made during the phase of developmental plasticity to optimise the phenotype for the probable environment of the mature organism, and epigenetic change is likely to be the mechanistic basis. Where there is a match between the predicted and actual mature environment, these responses are appropriate and assist survival. In contrast, inappropriate predictions increase the risk of disease. A key issue thus becomes the relative importance of early life events in informing intervention strategies during human development, rather than during adult life. Increasing awareness of the need to promote the health and nutrition of women of reproductive age is one important element for the prevention of osteoporotic fracture in future generations across the globe.

Acknowledgements We are grateful to the Medical Research Council; the Wellcome Trust, the Arthritis Research Campaign; the National Osteoporosis Society and the Cohen Trust for support of our research programme into the developmental origins of osteoporotic fracture. Dr. M K Javaid was in receipt of an ARC Clinical Research Fellowship. The manuscript was prepared by Mrs. G Strange.

References

Antoniades L, MacGregor AJ, Andrew T, et al. (2003). Association of birthweight with osteoporosis and osteoarthritis in adult twins. *Rheumatology* **42**: 791–796.

Barker DJP (1995). Fetal origins of coronary heart disease. *BMJ* **311**: 171–174.

Bateson P (2001). Fetal experience and good adult disease. *Int J Epidemiol* **30**: 928–934.

Consensus Development Conference (1991). Prophylaxis and treatment of osteoporosis. *Osteoporosis Int* **1**: 114–117.

Cooney CA, Dave AA, Wolff GL (2002). Maternal methyl supplements in mice affect epigenetic variation and DNA methylation of offspring. *J Nutr* **132**(Suppl 8): 2393S–2400S.

Cooper C (2003). Epidemiology of osteoporosis. In: Favus MJ (ed.), *Primer on the metabolic bone diseases and disorders of mineral metabolism*. 5th edition. Washington, DC: American Society for Bone and Mineral Research, pp. 307–313.

Cooper C, Cawley MID, Bhalla A, et al. (1995). Childhood growth, physical activity and peak bone mass in women. *J Bone Min Res* **10**: 940–947.

Cooper C, Fall C, Egger P, et al. (1997). Growth in infancy and bone mass in later life. *Ann Rheum Dis* **56**: 17–21.

Cooper C, Eriksson JG, Forsén T, et al. (2001). Maternal height, childhood growth and risk of hip fracture in later life: a longitudinal study. *Osteoporosis Int* **12**: 623–629.

Dennison E, Hindmarsh P, Fall C, et al. (1999). Profiles of endogenous circulating cortisol and bone mineral density in healthy elderly men. *J Clin Endocrinol Metab* **84**: 3058–3063.

Dennison EM, Arden NK, Keen RW, et al. (2001). Birthweight, vitamin D receptor genotype and the programming of osteoporosis. *Paediatr Peri Epidemiol* **15**: 211–219.

Dennison EM, Syddall HE, Rodriguez S, et al. (2004). Polymorphism in the growth hormone gene, weight in infancy, and adult bone mass. *J Clin Endocrinol Metab* **89**: 4898–4903.

Dennison EM, Syddall HE, Sayer AA, et al. (2005). Birth weight and weight at 1 year are independent determinants of bone mass in the seventh decade: the Hertfordshire cohort study. *Pediatr Res* **57**(4): 582–586.

Fall C, Hindmarsh P, Dennison E, et al. (1998). Programming of growth hormone secretion and bone mineral density in elderly men; an hypothesis. *J Clin Endocrinol Metab* **83**: 135–139.

Gluckman PD, Hanson MA (2004). Living with the past: evolution, development and patterns of disease. *Science* **305**: 1733–1736.

Godfrey K, Walker-Bone K, Robinson S, et al. (2001). Neonatal bone mass: influence of parental birthweight, maternal smoking, body composition, and activity during pregnancy. *J Bone Min Res* **16**: 1694–1703.

Javaid MK, Crozier SR, Harvey NC, Gale CR, Dennison EM, Boucher BJ, Arden NK, Godfrey KM, Cooer C, Princess Anne Hospital Study Group. (2006, Jan 7). Maternal vitamin D status during pregnancy and childhood bone mass at age 9 years: a longitudinal study. *Lancet* **367**(9504): 36–43. Erratum in: *Lancet* 2006, May 6; **367**(9521): 1486.

Keen R, Egger P, Fall C, et al. (1997). Polymorphisms of the vitamin D receptor, infant growth and adult bone mass. *Calcif Tiss Int* **60**: 233–235.

Lucas A (1991). Programming by early nutrition in man. In: Bock GR, Whelan J (eds.), *The childhood environment and adult disease*. New York: Wiley, pp. 38–55.

Phillips DIW, Barker DJP, Fall CHD, et al. (1998). Elevated plasma cortisol concentrations: a link between low birthweight and the insulin resistance syndrome? *J Clin Endocrinol Metab* **83**: 757–760.

Ralston SH (1998). Do genetic markers aid in risk assessment? *Osteoporosis Int* **8**: S37–S42.

Weaver IC, Cervoni N, Champagne FA, et al. (2004). Epigenetic programming by maternal behaviour. *Nat Neurosci* **7**: 847–854.

West-Eberhard MJ (2003). *Developmental plasticity and evolution*. 1st edition. New York: Oxford University Press.

Widdowson EM, McCance RA (1974). The determinants of growth and form. *Proceedings of the Royal Society of London* **185**: 1–17.

Zamora SA, Rizzoli R, Belli DC, et al. (1999). Vitamin D supplementation during infancy is associated with higher bone mineral mass in prepubertal girls. *J Clin Endocrinol Metab* **84**: 4541–4544.

Does Having Been Breastfed in Infancy Influence Lipid Profile in Later Life?: A Review of the Literature

Richard M. Martin and George Davey Smith

Abstract High plasma concentrations of cholesterol are a principal risk factor for atherogenesis and thus a major cause of cardiovascular disease. Animal and epidemiological evidence suggest that exposures acting in early life may play a role in cardiovascular disease risk, and infant nutrition is one early-life factor that has generated much interest amongst lifecourse researchers in recent years. A systematic review of epidemiological studies found that mean total cholesterol levels in adults were 0.18 mmol/L (95% CI = 0.06 to 0.30) lower amongst those who had been breastfed compared with those who received formula milk. Experimental evidence from the follow-up into adolescence of nutritional manipulation trials in preterm infants provides support for the hypothesis that breast milk may programme a beneficial lipid profile in later life. However, data in term infants are largely observational and so residual confounding can never be excluded, and there is little consistent evidence that any effect of breastfeeding on lipids translates into a reduced risk of cardiovascular disease in later life. The mechanistic basis for a programming effect of breastfeeding on adult cholesterol levels remains to be established in humans.

Keywords Infant nutrition • breastfeeding • cholesterol • cardiovascular disease • lifecourse • nutritional programming

Abbreviations CF: cow's milk formula; CVD: cardiovascular disease; FSR: fractional synthesis rate; HM: human milk; MCF: modified cow's milk formula

1 Importance

High plasma concentrations of cholesterol, in particular those of low-density lipoprotein (LDL) cholesterol, are one of the principal risk factors for the development of atherosclerotic plaques and thus a major cause of premature morbidity and mortality

R.M. Martin(✉) and G. Davey Smith
Department of Social Medicine, University of Bristol, Bristol, BS8 2PR
richard.martin@bristol.ac.uk

B. Koletzko et al. (eds.), *Early Nutrition Programming and Health Outcomes in Later Life: Obesity and Beyond*,

from heart attack, stroke and peripheral vascular disease. A number of lines of evidence support the idea that the pathogenesis of cardiovascular disease begins in early life. For example, in young USA combatants who were killed in action during the Korean War (mean age 22 years), autopsies revealed that 77% had some evidence of atherosclerosis and 15% had clinically significant narrowing of vessels (Enos et al. 1953). Similar results were published for Vietnam combat fatalities (McNamara et al. 1971). More recent autopsy studies based on male and female accidental deaths suggest that focal lipid accumulation begins in infancy and is present in over 60% of children around puberty (Stary 2000). In the Bogalusa Heart Study, atherosclerotic plaques were present in 8% of 2–15 year olds, rising to 69% at 26–39 years (Berenson et al. 1998). These data suggest that exposures acting in very early life may play an important role in the development of later cardiovascular disease.

Empirical evidence for a specific role of breastfeeding in infancy was suggested by the post-mortem studies of Osborn in 1967 (Osborn 1967). He interviewed the mothers of 109 deceased children and young adults (up to 20 years of age) and found that atherosclerosis on post-mortem occurred in 60% (25/42) of subjects who had been wholly artificially-fed, compared with 25% of subjects who had been breastfed (17/67). In line with Osborn's findings, an ecological study demonstrated that infant mortality rates from diarrhoea were correlated with coronary heart disease mortality rates in adulthood, amongst men (regression coefficient: 0.80) and women (regression coefficient: 0.63) born in 1917–1921 in 17 US Registration States (Buck and Simpson 1982). Since breastfeeding was strongly associated with mortality from diarrhoea in the past, the authors speculated that breastfeeding might be a common factor, protecting against both diarrhoea in infancy and, through some biological mechanism (such as the promotion of efficient metabolism of cholesterol), later cardiovascular mortality. Any primary prevention strategy based on infant nutrition is immensely appealing because of its inherent population-based focus and the potential for large public health benefits of even small shifts in the population distribution of cardiovascular disease risk factors (Rose 1985).

2 Evidence from Animal Studies

In a series of baboon experiments, Mott and McGill showed that juvenile baboons (70–90 weeks of age) that were breastfed as infants had lower serum cholesterol levels than those formula fed, primarily due to lower HDL cholesterol concentrations (Mott et al. 1995). There were no differences in LDL cholesterol levels. Juvenile baboons that had been breastfed had 44% higher hepatic LDL-receptor mRNA concentrations and a 25% lower bile acid synthetic rate than bottle-fed baboons, providing evidence that breastfeeding, compared with formula feeding, may imprint differences in cholesterol metabolism. Experiments on baboons also suggested that breastfeeding throughout infancy, followed by consumption of a high saturated fatty acid diet, increased later dyslipidaemia and the extent of atherosclerosis on necropsy at age 5 years compared with formula feeding, indicating that breastfeeding may interact adversely with a subsequent Western diet compared with formula feeding (Mott et al. 1982).

3 Systematic Reviews of Epidemiological Studies in Humans

In 2002, Owen et al. published a thorough meta-analysis of published studies on the association of having been breastfed with cholesterol levels that included 26 studies of the association in infancy (<1 year), 17 studies in which breastfeeding was related to cholesterol levels in children and adolescents (1–16 years) and 9 studies in adults (≥17 years) (Owen et al. 2002). In infancy, those who were breastfeeding had higher mean total cholesterol levels in 25 of 26 observations compared with those who were formula feeding (pooled mean difference: 0.64 mmol/L; 95% CI: 0.50 to 0.79) (Fig. 1), and higher LDL cholesterol levels in six of seven observations (mean difference: 0.57 mmol/L; 0.40 to 0.75). These findings are entirely consistent with the much greater concentration of cholesterol and LDL cholesterol in breast compared with modern formula milk.

Amongst children aged 1–16 years there was strong evidence of inconsistency in estimates between studies (p for heterogeneity = 0.01). The 95% confidence intervals of 16 of the 17 studies in this age group, however, all crossed the null value of no difference, including the largest study involving 4,023 subjects, and the pooled estimate from a random effects meta-analysis showed no difference in total cholesterol between breast and formula-fed infants (mean difference: 0.00 mol/L; −0.07 to 0.07) (Fig. 1). Similarly, LDL cholesterol levels were not related to breastfeeding in four studies in this age group (mean difference: 0.01 mol/L; −0.07 to 0.08; p for heterogeneity: 0.5).

In adults (≥17 years) mean total cholesterol levels were lower amongst those who were breastfed in seven of nine studies with no evidence of heterogeneity (p = 0.9), despite the wide age range (17–64 years) and range of birth dates (1920–1975).

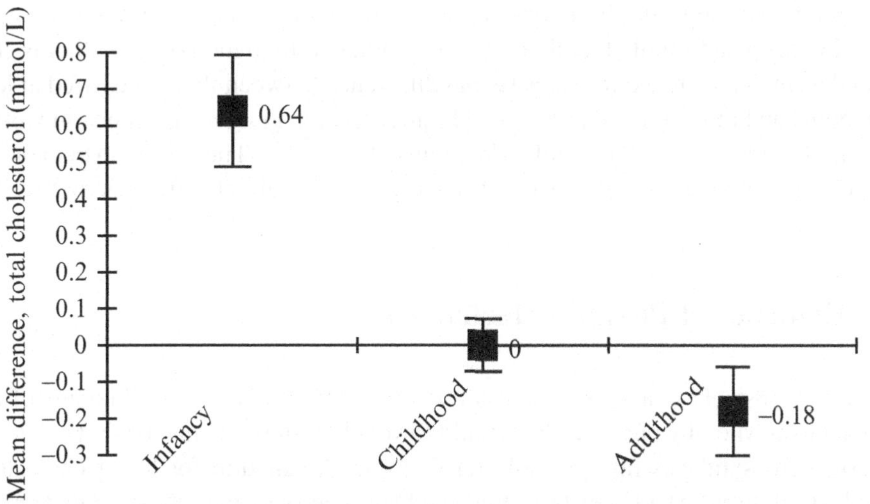

Fig. 1 Difference in mean total cholesterol levels in infants (<1 year), children (1–16 years) and adults (≥17 years) breastfed versus formula fed (Based on data presented in Owen et al. 2002)

For total cholesterol, the mean difference in those breastfed versus formula fed was –0.18 mmol/L (–0.30 to –0.06) (Fig. 1) and for LDL cholesterol it was –0.20 mmol/L (–0.32 to –0.08).

The apparent contradiction between a positive association of breastfeeding with cholesterol levels in infancy and a possible inverse association in adulthood suggested the possibility that the high cholesterol content of breastmilk compared with formula milk, leading to raised but reversible (on discontinuation) blood cholesterol levels, stimulates (programs) more efficient cholesterol metabolism in later life (Goedhart and Bindels 1994).

There are important sources of bias, however, that need to considered in the interpretation of this meta-analysis. Firstly, as the authors pointed out, publication bias is a possible explanation for the findings as there were fewer than 100 subjects in 67% of the observations and small studies may have been published only when they reported large effects. Secondly, inadequate control for confounding in individual studies is a possible explanation of the findings, though differences were reasonably consistent across eras, arguing against socioeconomic confounding since the relation between social class and infant feeding changed during the twentieth century. Finally, the impact of other aspects of study quality was not assessed and it is unclear to what extent the pooled associations were driven by poor quality studies.

While the positive association between breastfeeding and cholesterol levels in infancy appears robust, there are inconsistencies in the observational evidence relating breastfeeding with lipid profile in later life. Some authors suggest that prolonged breastfeeding (over 6 months [Strbak et al. 1993; Hromadova et al. 1997] or 12 months [Fall et al. 1992]) is associated with an atherogenic lipid profile and, as discussed above, in baboon experiments breastfeeding was associated with an atherogenic rather than beneficial lipid profile (McGill et al. 1996). Furthermore, studies published since the Owen review have been equivocal. Victora et al. (Victora et al. 2006) and Martin et al. (Martin et al. 2005), found very small and unimportant differences (in opposite directions) between infants who had been breastfed compared with those formula fed, though these studies were in men only. Williams et al. found a small difference in males (mean difference between those breastfed at least 6 months and those formula fed = –0.11 mmol/L) and a larger difference in women (mean difference = –0.42 mmol/L) (Williams et al. 2006). There was no evidence in the Owen meta-analysis, however, of heterogeneity in effect estimates by sex.

4 Evidence of Possible Mechanism

A further obstacle to assigning causality is the lack of evidence in humans of any mechanism whereby breastfeeding could lower cholesterol levels in adults. A lower endogenous synthesis rate of cholesterol is one explanation for lower cholesterol levels in adults who had been breastfed and Demmers et al. hypothesized that breastfed infants would have a lower fractional synthesis rate (FSR) (an index of hepatic cholesterol production) of cholesterol at 4 months, that would persist through to 18 months, when the diets of the infants would be similar (Demmers et al. 2005). A prospective partially randomised clinical trial was conducted between 1999–2002 with 47 infants, from their first week of life until 18 months of age, who received human milk (HM) exclusively until 6 months (n=15) or were randomized to receive modified cow's milk formula (MCF) with added cholesterol (n=15) or cow's milk formula (CF) (n=17) (with solids introduced to the MCF and CF diets at 4 months). The cholesterol contents of the HM, MCF, and CF diets were 120, 80, and 40 mg/L, respectively. FSR and plasma lipid levels were measured at 4 and 18 months. At 4 months, total cholesterol and LDL cholesterol levels were higher for infants fed HM and MCF, compared with CF. The FSR of endogenous cholesterol for the HM group was lower (P=0.017) at 4 months, compared with the CF group, while the endogenous cholesterol production of the MCF group was intermediate between those of the HM and CF fed infants. At 18 months, however, there were no differences between groups, suggesting that cholesterol synthesis in children aged 18 months is not programmed by exposure to the higher cholesterol levels found in human breastmilk. However, assessment at 18 months of age may be too early to see an effect, because differences in plasma lipid profiles between subjects breastfed and formula fed have not generally been seen until ≥17 years of age in observational studies (Owen et al. 2002).

5 Experimental Evidence in Humans

Most studies examining the association of breastfeeding in infancy with cholesterol levels in later life are observational and cannot exclude unmeasured or residual confounding by educational, socioeconomic and lifestyle factors associated with the mother's decision to breastfeed. Well conducted randomised controlled trials remove problems of confounding and selection bias, but randomization to breast- versus formula feeding is not feasible and may be unethical. However, randomisation has been feasible in special situations. Firstly, amongst preterm infants 20 years ago, banked breast milk from unrelated donors was commonly available and randomisation of infants to donor breast milk or formula was feasible and ethical (Singhal and Lucas 2004; Singhal et al. 2004). Secondly, a large randomised controlled trial of an intervention to promote breastfeeding exclusivity and duration, with analysis by "intention to treat" has been conducted, involving over 17,000 term and normal weight children in the Republic of Belarus who are now aged 11 years (PROBIT) (Kramer et al. 2001). These trials resulted in cohorts created by randomization, not the choice of the mother, enabling strong causal inferences with respect to breastfeeding effects on long-term outcomes.

The children in PROBIT are being followed-up for measurement of cardiovascular disease risk factors, including lipids. The randomised trial of different diets at birth in preterm infants, initiated by Alan Lucas in 1982, has provided unique data on the long-term effects of neonatal nutritional intake (Singhal and Lucas 2004;

Singhal et al. 2004). Two parallel randomised trials were conducted. The first allocated 502 preterm infants to either banked breast milk donated by unrelated lactating women or nutrient enriched preterm formula. Nutrient enriched formula provided 60% more energy and protein than banked breast milk or standard formula. The diets were randomly assigned in two strata – the trial diets alone and, in mothers who elected to express their own milk, the trial diets were assigned as a supplement to mother's milk. In analyses of the long term outcomes of infant feeding mode, the two strata have been combined. While there was considerable attrition at the 13–16 year follow-up – 130 (26%) of the original 502 infants were successfully followed up – there is little reason to think that the groups should be biased as equal efforts were made to trace the subjects regardless of trial allocation. In the second trial, standard term formula was compared with nutrient enriched preterm formula. As before, the allocated feed was assigned as a supplement amongst mothers who elected to express their own milk. 86 of the original 424 participants (20%) were followed-up into adolescence.

Results of lipid profiles at ages 13–16 years, comparing banked breastmilk versus preterm formula were published in 2004 (Singhal et al. 2004). The major finding was that the ratio LDL:HDL cholesterol was 14% lower in those randomised to banked breastmilk (mean difference = –0.34; 95% CI: –0.67 to –0.01) (Fig. 2). These differences remained after multivariable adjustment. An increased percent of enteral intake by volume consumed as human milk was associated with a reduced LDL:HDL ratio in a dose response manner (p for trend = 0.04), as well as lower apoB to apoA-1 (p = 0.004). The lipoprotein profile of the adolescents did not differ significantly between infants randomised to term formula compared with preterm formula and a greater proportion of pre-term formula intake was not associated with the LDL:HDL ratio (p for trend = 0.8). The authors concluded that

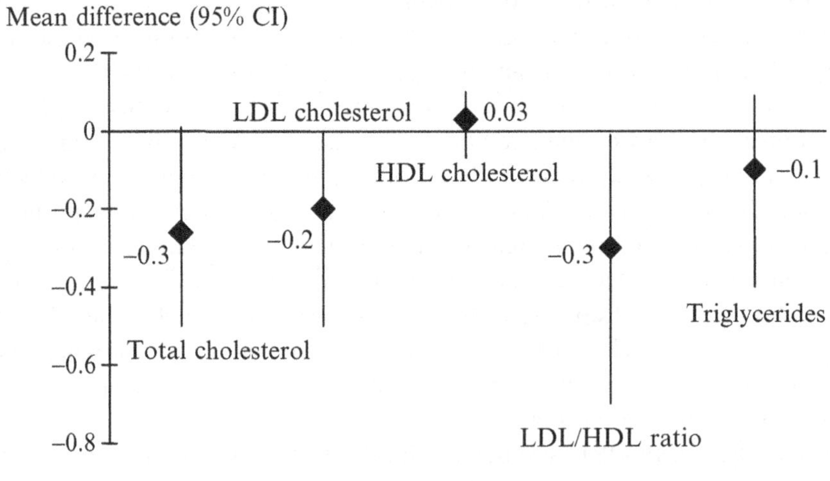

Fig. 2 Breast milk feeding and lipoprotein profile in adolescents born preterm: banked breast milk (n = 66) versus preterm formula (n = 64). Mean differences are presented (mmol/L) with 95% confidence intervals (CI) (Based on data presented in Singhal et al. 2004)

breast milk feeding had a dose-response beneficial effect on lipoprotein profile in adolescence.

In a secondary analysis, ignoring the randomisation, the authors showed that each 100 g increase in weight in the first 2 weeks of life resulted in an increase in LDL:HDL ratio of 0.2. Further, the difference in LDL:HDL ratio between those fed breast milk and those who were formula fed disappeared after adjustment for weight change in the first 2 weeks of life. The results of this secondary analysis, along with findings published from the preterm trials in relation to insulin and blood pressure, provided evidence for a new hypothesis about the early origins of cardiovascular disease, proposed by Singhal and Lucas, the growth acceleration hypothesis (Singhal and Lucas 2004). This hypothesis suggests that that faster early growth, as a result of a nutrient enriched diet, adversely programmes the principal components of the metabolic syndrome (vice versa for breastfeeding). Data from other large cohorts, such as PROBIT, are now required to confirm or refute this hypothesis.

6 Clinical Events

The public health importance of these findings rests on their translation into benefit on clinical outcomes. If breastfeeding did lower cholesterol in adulthood, a reduction in later cardiovascular disease (CVD) incidence would be expected. We have updated our previously published meta-analysis investigating the association between having been breastfed and CVD mortality (Martin et al. 2004a). This analysis involves five studies (Fall et al. 1992; Wingard et al. 1994; Rich-Edwards et al. 2004; Martin et al. 2004a, 2005) (with seven estimates because two studies showed sex specific results) (Fig. 3). The pooled data are relatively consistent in suggesting that breastfeeding does not have an important role in protecting against future cardiovascular disease or coronary heart disease risk. Furthermore, prolonged breastfeeding for over 9–12 months was not associated with cardiovascular disease (pooled rate ratio for breastfed >9–12 months vs. never breastfed: 1.03; 95% CI: 0.92–1.15; $I^2=4\%$) or coronary heart disease (pooled rate ratio for breastfed >9–12 months vs. never breastfed: 0.95; 95% CI: 0.83–1.10; $I^2=0\%$).

7 Conclusion

Observational studies suggest that breastfeeding in infancy is associated with a small reduction in total and LDL cholesterol in adulthood. A trial of preterm infants provides experimental evidence in support of the hypothesis (Singhal et al. 2004). There is currently no evidence, however, that any potential effect of breastfeeding on lipid profile translates into a reduction in risk of CVD in later life (Martin et al. 2004a). Further, there is not yet any convincing mechanistic basis

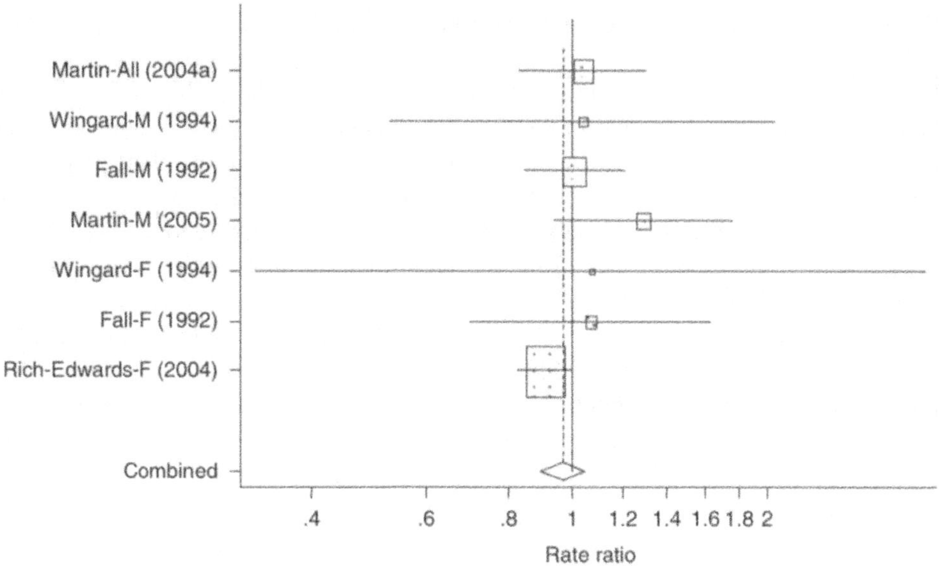

Fig. 3 Pooled rate ratio (95% CI) for CVD comparing infants who were ever breastfed versus infants who were never breastfed fed. The surname of the first author, the sex of the study participants (All = both male and female, F = female, M = male), is indicated on the y axis. The box area for each study is proportional to the inverse of the variance, with horizontal lines showing the 95% confidence intervals. The combined estimate is based on a random effects model shown by the dashed vertical line and diamond (95% CI). The solid vertical line represents the null result, i.e., rate ratio = 1. Pooled rate ratio: 0.97 (0.90–1.05); p = 0.4. Test for heterogeneity: Q = 5.643 on six degrees of freedom (p = 0.5). I^2 (% variation attributable to heterogeneity) = 0%

for a programming effect of breastfeeding on adult lipid profile (Demmers et al. 2005). The long-term benefits of breastfeeding will be hard to demonstrate convincingly in observational studies because of the strong social patterning of this exposure and the problems of recall bias, maintaining high rates of follow-up and adequate control for confounding in long-term studies (Davey Smith and Ebrahim 2002). Large long-term birth cohort studies with detailed prospective measures of breastfeeding exclusivity and duration (Martin et al. 2004b), comprehensive data on potential confounding factors, as well as the inclusion of unpublished data within systematic meta-analyses (Owen et al. 2003) may offer some reassurance against biased results. The most robust evidence comes from randomized controlled trials. The hypothesis that breastfeeding influences later CVD risk factors in term infants could ethically and feasibly be tested on an intention-to-treat basis, in large, controlled trials of successful breastfeeding promotion interventions with a record of high rates of follow-up, the best example of which is perhaps the PROBIT study. This study is currently being followed up with funding from the European Union, the Canadian Institutes of Health Research (CIHR), and the National Institutes of Health (NIH).

Acknowledgements The PROBIT study is currently being followed up with funding from the: European Communities specific Research and Technology Development program "Early Nutrition Programming for Adult Health" Project: EARly Nutrition programming-long term follow up of Efficacy and Safety Trials and integrated epidemiological, genetic, animal, consumer and economic research (EARNEST), grant number FOOD-CT-2005-007036; the Canadian Institutes of Health Research (CIHR); and the National Institutes of Health (NIH), grant number 1R01HD050758-01A2.

References

Berenson, G.S., Srinivasan, S.R., Bao, W., Newman, III, W.P., Tracy, R.E., Wattigney, W.A., & Bogalusa Heart Study (1998) Association between multiple cardiovascular risk factors and atherosclerosis in children and young adults. *N Engl J Med* **338**, 1650–1656.

Buck, C. & Simpson, H. (1982) Infant diarrhoea and subsequent mortality from heart disease and cancer. *J Epidemiol Community Health* **36**, 27–30.

Davey Smith, G. & Ebrahim, S. (2002) Data dredging, bias, or confounding. *BMJ* **325**, 1437–1438.

Demmers, T.A., Jones, P.J.H., Wang, Y., Krug, S., Creutzinger, V., & Heubi, J.E. (2005) Effects of early cholesterol intake on cholesterol biosynthesis and plasma lipids among infants until 18 months of age. *Pediatrics* **115**, 1594–1601.

Enos, W.F., Holmes, R.H., & Beyer, J. (1953) Coronary disease among United States soldiers killed in action in Korea. *JAMA* **152**, 1090–1093.

Fall, C.H.D., Barker, D.J.P., Osmond, C., Winter, P.D., Clark, P.M.S., & Hales, C.N. (1992) Relation of infant feeding to adult serum cholesterol concentration and death from ischaemic heart disease. *BMJ* **304**, 801–805.

Goedhart, A.C. & Bindels, J.G. (1994) The composition of human milk as a model for the design of infant formulas: recent findings and possible applications. *Nutr Res Rev* **7**, 1–23.

Hromadova, M., Kostalova, L., Leskova, L., & Kapellerova, A. (1997) Relationship between the duration of the breastfeeding period and the lipoprotein profile of children at the age of 13 years. *Physiol Res* **46**, 21–25.

Kramer, M.S., Chalmers, B., Hodnett, E.D., Sevkovskaya, Z., Dzikovich, I., Shapiro, S., Collet, J.P., Vanilovich, I., Mezen, I., Ducruet, T., Shishko, G., Zubovich, V., Mknuik, D., Gluchanina, E., Dombrovskiy, V., Ustinovitch, A., Kot, T., Bogdanovich, N., Ovchinikova, L., Helsing, E., & PROBIT Study Group (Promotion of Breastfeeding Intervention Trial) (2001) Promotion of Breastfeeding Intervention Trial (PROBIT): a randomized trial in the Republic of Belarus. *JAMA* **285**, 413–420.

Martin, R.M., Davey Smith, G., Tilling, K., Frankel, S., & Gunnell, D. (2004a) Breastfeeding and cardiovascular mortality: the Boyd Orr cohort and a systematic review with meta-analysis. *Eur Heart J* **25**, 778–786.

Martin, R.M., Ness, A.R., Gunnell, D., Emmett, P.M., & Davey Smith, G. (2004b) Does breastfeeding in infancy lower blood pressure in childhood? The Avon Longitudinal Study of Parents and Children. *Circulation* **109**, 1259–1266.

Martin, R.M., Ben-Shlomo, Y., Gunnell, D., Elwood, P., Yarnell, J.W.G., & Davey Smith, G. (2005) Breast feeding and cardiovascular disease risk factors, incidence, and mortality: the Caerphilly study. *J Epidemiol Community Health* **59**, 121–129.

McGill, H.C., Jr., Mott, G.E., Lewis, D.S., McMahan, C.A., & Jackson, E.M. (1996) Early determinants of adult metabolic regulation: effects of infant nutrition on adult lipid and lipoprotein metabolism. *Nutr Rev* **54**, S31–S40.

McNamara, M.J.J., Molot, M.M., Stremple, M.J., & Cutting, C.R. (1971) Coronary artery disease in combat casualties in Vietnam. *J Am Med Assoc* **216**, 1185–1187.

Mott, G.E., McMahan, C.A., Kelley, J.L., Farley, C.M., & McGill, H.C. (1982) Influence of infant and juvenile diets on serum cholesterol, lipoprotein cholesterol, and apolipoprotein concentrations in juvenile baboons (Papio sp.). *Atherosclerosis* **45**, 191–202.

Mott, G.E., Jackson, E.M., DeLallo, L., Lewis, D.S., & McMahan, C.A. (1995) Differences in cholesterol metabolism in juvenile baboons are programmed by breast- versus formula-feeding. *J Lipid Res* **36**, 299–307.

Osborn, G.R. (1967) Stages in development of coronary disease observed from 1500 young subjects: relationship of hypotension and infant feeding to aetiology. *Colloq Int CNRS* **169**, 93–139.

Owen, C.G., Whincup, P.H., Odoki, K., Gilg, J.A., & Cook, D.G. (2002) Infant feeding and blood cholesterol: a study in adolescents and a systematic review. *Pediatrics* **110**, 597–608.

Owen, C.G., Whincup, P.H., Gilg, J.A., & Cook, D.G. (2003) Effect of breast feeding in infancy on blood pressure in later life: systematic review and meta-analysis. *BMJ* **327**, 1189–1195.

Rich-Edwards, J.W., Stampfer, M.J., Manson, J.E., Rosner, B., Hu, F.B., Michels, K.B., & Willett, W. (2004) Breastfeeding during infancy and the risk of cardiovascular disease in adulthood. *Epidemiology* **15**, 550–556.

Rose, G. (1985) Sick individuals and sick populations. *Int J Epidemiol* **14**, 32–38.

Singhal, A. & Lucas, A. (2004) Early origins of cardiovascular disease: is there a unifying hypothesis? *Lancet* **363**, 1642–1645.

Singhal, A., Cole, T.J., Fewtrell, M., & Lucas, A. (2004) Breastmilk feeding and lipoprotein profile in adolescents born preterm: follow-up of a prospective randomised study. *Lancet* **363**, 1571–1578.

Stary, H.C. (2000) Lipid and macrophage accumulations in arteries of children and the development of atherosclerosis. *Am J Clin Nutr* **72**, 1297S–1306S.

Strbak, V., Hromadova, M., Kostalova, L., & Kapellerova, A. (1993) Search for optimal age for weaning. Ten year prospective study. *Endocrinol Regul* **27**, 215–221.

Victora, C.G., Horta, B.L., Post, P., Lima, R.C., De Leon Elizalde, J.W., Gerson, B.M.C., & Barros, F.C. (2006) Breast feeding and blood lipid concentrations in male Brazilian adolescents. *J Epidemiol Community Health* **60**, 621–625.

Williams, M.J.A., Williams, S.M., & Poulton, R. (2006) Breast feeding is related to C reactive protein concentration in adult women. *J Epidemiol Community Health* **60**, 146–148.

Wingard, D.L., Criqui, M.H., Edelstein, S.L., Tucker, J., Tomlinson-Keasey, C., Schwartz, J.E., & Friedman, H.S. (1994) Is breast-feeding associated with adult longevity? *Am J Public Health* **84**, 1458–1462.

The Early Origins of Atherosclerosis

Atul Singhal

Abstract Atherosclerosis has a long pre-clinical phase with development of pathological changes in arteries of children and young adults decades before overt clinical manifestations of disease. Nutritional factors in both infancy and childhood have been shown to be important in this process and affect lifetime cardiovascular disease risk. Breast-feeding in particular is associated with benefits for long-term cardiovascular risk factors possibly as a consequence of a slower pattern of growth in breast-fed compared to formula-fed infants. In fact, the benefits of slower growth for later health and longevity, appears to be a fundamental biological phenomenon conserved across diverse animal species. The nutritional programming of atherosclerosis could therefore be regarded as a specific example of programming of human ageing as seen previously in programming of lifespan and telomere length in animals. The critical window for these effects is unknown, but evidence is accumulating for programming effects of growth from very early in infancy.

Keywords Breast-feeding • cardiovascular disease • growth acceleration • programming

Abbreviations CVD: cardiovascular disease; FMD: flow-mediated dilation; IGF-1: insulin-like growth factor 1

1 Introduction

Atherosclerotic cardiovascular disease (CVD) is the leading cause of death and disability, and the most important public health priority in the West (British Heart Foundation 2004). Yet, despite great progress in its clinical management, the prevalence of CVD continues to increase. In the UK alone an estimated 2.7 million

A. Singhal
The MRC Childhood Nutrition Research Centre, Institute of Child Health,
30 Guilford Street, London, UK
a.singhal@ich.ucl.ac.uk

B. Koletzko et al. (eds.), *Early Nutrition Programming and Health Outcomes in Later Life: Obesity and Beyond*,

people are now living with coronary heart disease – a number that has risen sharply. Consequently, the role of prevention has become a major priority for public health policy and future scientific research. This review considers the evidence that atherosclerosis begins in childhood and that early nutritional factors have the potential to reduce lifetime cardiovascular risk.

2 The Childhood Origins of Atherosclerosis

Autopsy studies showing atherosclerotic changes in the coronary arteries of solders killed in the Korean and Vietnamese wars first identified the presence of atherosclerosis in the young and stimulated research into mechanisms that regulate its early development. Similar studies in children, particularly from the Bogalusa Heart Study, demonstrated a high prevalence of coronary atherosclerosis by the third decade of life (Berenson et al. 1998). The presence and extent of atherosclerotic lesions in these reports correlated positively with established cardiovascular risk factors, such as lipoprotein profile, blood pressure, and body mass index. Importantly, the severity of pathological lesions was associated with an increase in number of risk factors, in accordance with the Framingham risk score for predicting cardiovascular mortality in adults. These autopsy findings have now been confirmed in other populations and extended to atherosclerosis at different vascular sites.

It is now accepted that atherosclerosis has a long pre-clinical phase with development of pathological changes in arteries of children decades before overt clinical manifestations of disease. Nutritional factors in childhood have been shown to be particularly important in this process and have a major impact on conventional cardiovascular risk factors that affect vascular health and lifetime CVD risk (Berenson et al. 1998). These factors track into adulthood and have a strong, independent influence on CVD risk. Obesity in children, for instance, affects adult cardiovascular health, independently of risk factors in adults (Falkstedt et al. 2007). The estimated public health impact is large. In fact, it has been suggested that the current increase in childhood obesity will reverse the recent improvements in morbidity and lifespan achieved through control of CVD risk factors in adulthood (Olshansky et al. 2005). Attention to nutrition throughout the life course (and not just in adults) is therefore important in preventing CVD. Consequently, the American Heart and American Pediatric Associations have both targeted children for nutritional interventions aimed at primary prevention of CVD (Kavey et al. 2003).

Other than effects on classical cardiovascular risk factors, nutrition in childhood also has direct effects on vascular biology associated with the early atherosclerotic process. These changes can now be detected non-invasively in children using vascular ultrasound. Arterial distensibility, for instance, a measure of arterial wall elasticity or compliance which is known to correlate closely with CVD risk factors and extent of disease, is closely related to lipid profile and hence nutrition in adolescents. In fact, high cholesterol concentration has been associated with impaired brachial arterial distensibility in healthy children from as early as the first decade of life (Leeson et al. 2000).

Overall, there is now strong evidence to support the hypothesis that nutrition in childhood has a major impact on atherosclerotic disease. However, in terms of effect size, nutrition earlier in the life course, in fetal life and infancy, could make a greater contribution to lifetime CVD risk. Perinatal nutrition is therefore emerging as a major focus for programming research.

3 Nutritional Programming of Atherosclerosis

The concept that nutrition in infancy can have a long-term effect on, or programme, risk factors for CVD first emerged in the 1960s with the pioneering work of McCance. He showed that rats raised in small litters, and therefore overfed early in postnatal life, were programmed for greater body size as adults (McCance 1962). Subsequently, rats overfed in the brief suckling period were shown to have permanently higher plasma insulin and cholesterol concentrations while early nutrition in baboons was found to influence later obesity and atherosclerosis. In baboons, the effects of over-feeding in infancy for obesity emerged only after adolescence, demonstrating the later manifestation of these effects.

3.1 Birth Weight

In humans, several groups have shown that low birth weight, possibly as a result of reduced fetal growth and nutrition, is related to an increased risk of later CVD ('the fetal origins of adult disease hypothesis') (Barker 1995). Of relevance to the development of vascular disease, low birth weight was associated with sub-clinical measures of atherosclerosis such as impaired endothelial function and arterial distensibility in children. Further support for an intra-uterine effect on atherosclerosis emerged from studies which showed that maternal hypercholesterolemia was associated in the offspring with greatly increased fatty streak formation in infancy and accelerated progression of atherosclerosis during childhood (Palinski and Napoli 2002). However, a major limitation of these earlier studies is a lack of experimental evidence for a causal link between intra-uterine factors and later vascular health.

3.2 Breast-Feeding

The major focus of programming research in the post-natal period has been the impact of breast-feeding. Since the early studies in the 1960s (Osborne 1963) most, but not all reports have suggested that breast-fed infants have a lower risk of CVD, obesity, high cholesterol concentration, type II diabetes and high blood pressure. These observational data could be confounded by socio-economic and demographic differences between breast-fed and formula fed groups. In preterm infants, however, a causal association was testable using an experimental approach. Infants whose mothers decided not to breast-feed were randomly assigned to breast-milk donated by unrelated lactating mothers or to formula milk. Infants assigned to human milk versus formula, for an average of 4 weeks, were found to have marked benefits up to 16 years later for the major components of the metabolic syndrome (blood pressure, leptin 'resistance' suggestive of future obesity, insulin resistance and lipid profile) (Singhal and Lucas 2004). As further evidence of causation there were clear dose–response associations between the volume of breast-milk intake and later cardiovascular benefit (Singhal and Lucas 2004).

The effect size for beast-milk feeding on later CVD risk factors was substantial (Singhal and Lucas 2004). For blood pressure, for instance, a 3 mm Hg lower diastolic blood pressure in infants given breast-milk compared to formula has major public health implications and represents an effect greater than other non-pharmacological means of reducing blood pressure (such as weight loss, salt restriction, or exercise). Lowering population-wide diastolic blood pressure by only 2 mm Hg has been estimated to reduce the prevalence of hypertension by 17%, the risk of coronary heart disease by 6% and the risk of stroke/transient ischaemic attacks by 15%. Such an intervention would be expected to prevent an estimated 100,000 cardiovascular events annually among those aged 35–64, in the USA alone. Similarly, the 10% lowering of cholesterol concentration with breast-feeding compares favourably with the effects of dietary interventions in adults, which lower cholesterol by only 3–6%. Such an effect on cholesterol concentration would be expected to reduce the incidence of cardiovascular disease by approximately 25% and mortality by 13–14%.

4 Early Growth and Later Atherosclerotic Risk

Understanding the mechanisms by which breast-feeding affects long-term CVD risk could help in the primary prevention of atherosclerosis and also in the development of preventative strategies for formula-fed infants. The most common explanation, confounding by socio-biological factors that influence both the mothers' decision to breast-feed and later cardiovascular risk, is unlikely in view of the experimental evidence from preterm infants. Other potential explanations include the long-term health benefits of specific nutrients in breast-milk, which are absent from some formulas – such as effects of long-chain polyunsaturated fatty acids in lowering later blood pressure. Most recently, we have suggested that the cardiovascular advantages of breast-feeding may be due to slower growth in breast-fed versus formula-fed infants – the growth acceleration hypothesis.

4.1 Studies in Pre-term Infants

The postnatal growth acceleration hypothesis suggests that faster growth (upward centile crossing) particularly in infancy adversely programmes the metabolic syndrome (Singhal and Lucas 2004). Consistent with this, faster neonatal growth was shown to programme insulin resistance and endothelial dysfunction (which has a central role in the initiation and progression of atherosclerosis and can be measured non-invasively using vascular ultrasound as the vasodilatator response to increased blood flow (flow-mediated dilation, or FMD). As suggested by the fetal origins hypothesis, we found that low birth weight was associated with lower FMD 13–16 years later. However, as shown previously for insulin resistance, the effect of low birth weight on vascular function was displaced by adverse effects of faster post-natal weight gain (Singhal et al. 2004). Because small babies tend to show faster post-natal growth, these analyses suggested that early post-natal growth could contribute to the association between low birth weight and later CVD risk (Singhal and Lucas 2004). The size of the effect was substantial. Adolescents with the greatest weight gain in the first 2 weeks of life had 4% lower FMD of the brachial artery than those with the lowest weight gain: an effect similar to that of insulin dependent diabetes mellitus (4%) and smoking (6%) in adults. Importantly, similar adverse effects on vascular health were observed for faster linear growth in the first few weeks of life (Singhal et al. 2004).

4.2 Studies in Term Infants

The programming effects of growth in infancy are not confined to infants born prematurely. In an intervention study of infants born full-term, but small for gestation, those randomly assigned to a standard formula for the first 9 months had lower blood pressure 6–8 years later than infants fed a nutrient-enriched formula that promoted growth (Singhal et al. 2007). Further analysis suggested that faster growth explained the adverse effects of a nutrient-enriched formula on later blood pressure. Similar observations were observed for adiposity; infants randomised to the high protein formula had greater adiposity later in life, an effect explained by their faster growth rate (A. Singhal 2007). Interestingly, the adverse effects of faster growth were seen in both breast-fed and formula-fed infants.

Studies in healthy full term infants also support the programming effects of growth in infancy. Faster growth has been linked with higher blood pressure (now seen in more than five studies, as reviewed recently; Singhal et al. 2007), insulin resistance and, in three systematic reviews (in >21 studies) obesity later in life (Ong and Loos 2006). These data include effects of faster weight gain in programming greater blood pressure and adiposity in approximately 5,000 healthy children born at term from Avon Longitudinal Study of Parents and Children, most of whom were breast-fed (Charakida et al. 2006). The growth acceleration concept therefore challenges current practices often aimed at maximising growth in infancy.

4.3 Animal Studies

Data from studies in animals strongly support the adverse effects of faster early growth and a higher plane of postnatal nutrition in programming the metabolic syndrome (McCance 1962; Ozanne and Hales 2004). In fact the adverse long-term effects of faster early growth emerge as a fundamental biological phenomenon across animal species (Metcalfe and Monaghan 2001). On the other hand, restriction of growth and nutrition during critical windows in development may have favourable programming effects, as first suggested from as early as the 1930s for lifespan in rats and now seen for adiposity, and lifespan in numerous animal species as diverse as mice, flies, worms and even yeast (Rollo 2002; Longo and Finch 2003). It appears, therefore, that research into the early origins of both aging and CVD could reflect similar underlying mechanisms affecting cellular senescence – i.e. the impact of early growth and nutrition, via programming of hormonal systems such as insulin and insulin-like growth factor 1 (IGF-1) (which are conserved throughout these species) (Longo and Finch 2003) on adult degenerative processes. Atherosclerosis could result from accelerated biological aging as suggested recently by data showing a greater risk of CVD in men who had shorter leukocyte telomeres, a marker of cellular senescence (Brouilette et al. 2007). The nutritional programming of CVD could, therefore, be regarded as a specific instance of programming of human ageing as seen previously in studies of lifespan and telomere length in animals (Ozanne and Hales 2004). The common mechanism of accelerated aging could also explain the wide ranging effects of nutritional programming on diverse physiological systems that effect CVD risk.

4.4 When Is the Critical Window?

We suggested that early infancy, a time of the fastest growth rate, is likely to be a particularly sensitive window for nutrition programming (Singhal and Lucas 2004). In the 1960s the critical window for programming effects in animal studies was suggested to be as early as the first 5 postnatal days (Dubos et al. 1966). Consistent with this, faster growth in the first few weeks (regardless of gestation or birth weight), has now been associated with later insulin resistance and endothelial function (Singhal and Lucas 2004), the development of adult obesity in a US cohort (Stettler et al. 2005), programming of IGF-1 concentration, and in unpublished data, for later blood pressure and endothelial function in twins born at term, and for adiposity in adults born preterm (A. Singhal 2007). However, the data are inconsistent with some studies showing that faster weight gain in childhood rather than infancy increased later CVD risk (Barker et al. 2005).

5 Conclusions

Whilst further research is needed to define the critical windows for nutritional programming, the concept that growth and nutrition have a major impact on CVD risk, is now firmly established. These early factors interact with subsequent environment to predispose to rather than directly cause later atherosclerotic disease. Nevertheless, given the exposure to 'atherogenic' environments of many populations from both the West and developing countries, nutritional programming is likely to have a substantial effect on CVD, and hence public health, world-wide.

References

Barker DJ (1995). Fetal origins of coronary heart disease. *BMJ* **311**: 171–174.

Barker DJP, Osmond C, Forsen TJ, Kajantie E, Eriksson JG (2005). Trajectories of growth among children who have coronary events as adults. *N Engl J Med* **353**: 1802–1809.

Berenson GS, Srinivasan SR, Nicklas TA (1998). 'Atherosclerosis: a nutritional disease of childhood. *Am J Cardiol* **82**: 22T–29T.

British Heart Foundation (2004). Compendium of annual statistics.; www.heartstats.org

Brouilette SW, Moore JS, McMahon AD, Thompson JR, Ford I, Shepherd J, Packard CJ, Samani NJ (2007). Telomere length, risk of coronary heart disease, and statin treatment in the West of Scotland Primary Prevention Study: a nested case control study. *Lancet* **369**: 107–114.

Charakida M, Donald A, Singhal A, Halcox J, Ness A, Davey Smith G, Deanfield J (2006). Accelerated early postnatal growth is associated with increased blood pressure and body mass index in childhood. *Circulation* **114** (Suppl): 358a.

Dubos R, Savage D, Schaedler R (1966). Biological Freudianism: lasting effects of early environmental influences. *Paediatrics* **38**: 789–800. Reprinted in *Int J Epidemiol* 2005; **34**: 5–12.

Falkstedt D, Hemmingsson T, Rasmussen F, Lundberg I (2007). Body mass index in late adolescence and its association with coronary heart disease and stroke in middle age among Swedish men. *Int J Obes* **31**: 777–783.

Kavey RE, Daniels SR, Lauer RM, Atkins DL, Hayman LL, Taubert K (2003). American heart association guidelines for primary prevention of atherosclerotic cardiovascular disease beginning in childhood. *Circulation* **107**: 1562–1566.

Leeson CP, Whincup PH, Cook DG, Mullen MJ, Donald AE, Seymour CA, Deanfield JE (2000). 'Cholesterol and arterial distensibility in the first decade of life: a population-based study. *Circulation* **101**: 1533–1538.

Longo VD, Finch CE (2003). Evolutionary medicine: from dwarf model systems to healthy centenarians? *Science* **299**: 1342–1346.

McCance RA (1962). Food, growth and time. *Lancet* **2**: 671–676.

Metcalfe NB, Monaghan P (2001). Compensation for a bad start: grow now, pay later? *Trends Ecol Evol* **16**: 254–260.

Olshansky SJ, Passaro DJ, Hershow RC, Layden J, Carnes BA, Brody J, Hayflick L, Butler RN, Allison DB, Ludwig DS (2005). A potential decline in life expectancy in the United States in the 21st century. *N Engl J Med* **352**: 1138–1145.

Ong KK, Loos RJ (2006). Rapid infancy weight gain and subsequent obesity: systematic reviews and hopeful suggestions. *Acta Paediatr* **95**: 904–908.

Osborne GR (1963). The incubation period of coronary thrombosis. Butterworths, London.

Ozanne SE, Hales CN (2004). Catch-up growth and obesity in male mice. *Nature* **427**: 411–412.

Palinski W, Napoli C (2002). The fetal origins of atherosclerosis: maternal hypercholesterolemia, and cholesterol-lowering or antioxidant treatment during pregnancy influence in utero programming and postnatal susceptibility to atherogenesis. *FASEB J* **16**: 1348–1360.
Rollo CD (2002). Growth negatively impacts the life span of mammals. *Evol Dev* **4**: 55–61.
Singhal A, Lucas A (2004). Early origins of cardiovascular disease: is there a unifying hypothesis? *Lancet* **363**: 1642–1645.
Singhal A, Cole TJ, Fewtrell MS, Deanfield J, Lucas A (2004). Is slower early growth beneficial for long-term cardiovascular health? *Circulation* **109**: 1108–1113.
Singhal A, Cole TJ, Fewtrell M, Kennedy K, Stephenson T, Elias-Jones A, Lucas A (2007). Promotion of faster weight gain in infants born small for gestational age: is there an adverse effect on later blood pressure? *Circulation* **115**: 213–220.
Stettler N, Stallings VA, Troxel AB, Zhao J, Schinnar R, Nelson SE, Ziegler EE, Strom BL (2005). Weight gain in the first week of life and overweight in adulthood. A cohort study of European American subjects fed infant formula. *Circulation* **111**: 1897–1903.

Do LCPUFAs Influence Cardiovascular Function in Early Childhood?

J. Stewart Forsyth

Abstract In recent years there have been reports linking breast milk intake in infancy to lower blood pressure during childhood. The mechanisms underlying the relationship remain uncertain however there has been recent interest in the role of long chain polyunsaturated fatty acids (LCPUFAs). Several studies involving human adults have reported a lowering of blood pressure with n-3 fatty acid supplementation. Data relating to children are limited: however, two published randomised controlled studies report that LCPUFA supplementation in infancy may be associated with lower blood pressure in early childhood.

Keywords Infant feeding • LCPUFAs • blood pressure

Abbreviations ACTH: adrenocorticotrophic hormone; DHA: docosahexanenoic acid; EPA: eicosapentaenoic acid; LCPUFA: long chain polyunsaturated fatty acids

1 Introduction

In recent years there have been reports linking breast milk intake in infancy to lower blood pressure during childhood (Wilson et al. 1998; Taittonen et al. 1996; Singhal et al. 2001). Two longitudinal observational studies in term infants demonstrated that children who were breast fed for at least 3 months had lower systolic and diastolic blood pressures during later childhood and adolescence compared to children who were formula fed. This difference persisted after adjustments were made for known confounding variables (Wilson et al. 1998; Taittonen et al. 1996). In a trial involving preterm infants, children at age 15 years who had been randomised to banked breast milk had lower systolic and diastolic blood pressures

J.S. Forsyth
Ninewells Hospital and Medical School, Dundee, Scotland
stewartforsyth@nhs.net

B. Koletzko et al. (eds.), *Early Nutrition Programming and Health Outcomes in Later Life: Obesity and Beyond*,

compared to children who had received term or preterm formula in the newborn period (Singhal et al. 2001).

The mechanisms underlying the relationship of breast feeding to childhood blood pressure remain uncertain. In the preterm study there was no difference in blood pressure between infants receiving a term formula and infants who were fed a preterm formula, the latter containing additional protein, energy and minerals including sodium (Singhal et al. 2001). Breast milk contains a wide range of factors which are not included in formula milks and which may influence blood pressure, including trophic substances, hormones and specific nutrients.

2 Evidence for a Role for LCPUFAs

In recent years there has been considerable interest in the role of long chain polyunsaturated fatty acids (LCPUFAs) as these fatty acids are present in breast milk but were not routinely available in formula milks (Koletzko et al. 2001). These fatty acids are preferentially incorporated into neural cell membranes, and therefore studies have predominantly focused on their influence on visual and cognitive development (Makrides et al. 2000; Willatts et al. 1998). During the first weeks of life, preterm infants and some term infants, may not be able to synthesise sufficient LCPUFAs to meet demand, and therefore unsupplemented formula fed infants may experience a relative deficiency of LCPUFAs compared to breast fed infants (Cunnane et al. 2000).

It is also known that LCPUFAs are incorporated into other cell membranes including vascular endothelium (Engler et al. 1999b). Several studies in adults have reported a lowering of blood pressure with n-3 fatty acid supplementation (Mori and Beilin 2001; Mori et al. 1999), however there were no published studies relating LCPUFA supplementation to blood pressure in children.

As a follow-up to a previous study, in which we randomly assigned newborn infants to a formula with LCPUFAs or to a formula that was devoid of LCPUFAs but otherwise nutritionally similar (Forsyth et al. 1999) we investigated the relationship of LCPUFA supplementation in infancy to later childhood blood pressure (Forsyth et al. 2003). At the age of 6 years, the diastolic blood pressure was significantly lower in the children who had received LCPUFA supplementation in infancy compared to children who were fed the unsupplemented formula (57.3 vs. 60.9; mean difference −3.6 (CI −6.5 to −0.6); $p = 0.018$). There was a similar trend for systolic blood pressure but this was not significant. However, the mean blood pressure was significantly lower in the LCPUFA supplemented group. The reference breast fed group had similar blood pressures to the supplemented group.

More recently, a study involving supplementation of healthy 9 month old infants with 5 ml of fish oil or no fish oil for 3 months demonstrated a lower systolic blood pressure in infants who had received the fish oil supplementation. (Damsgaard et al. 2006) Interestingly though, a study involving maternal supplementation with fish oil during the first 4 months of lactation had no effect on blood pressure of the infant at age 2.5 years (Larnkjaer et al. 2006; Ulbak et al. 2004). Larnkjaer et al. (2006) also reported that there was no significant relationship between maternal fish oil supplementation and infant heart rate variability.

3 Possible Mechanisms

The mechanisms underlying the relationship of LCPUFAs to blood pressure remain speculative. In our study, the composition of trial formulas only differed significantly in the content of docosahexanenoic acid (DHA) and arachidonic acid. Several studies involving hypertensive adults have demonstrated a fall in blood pressure with an increased dietary intake of omega 3 fatty acids (Mori and Beilin 2001). In a double-blind, placebo controlled trial, Mori et al. (1999) showed that DHA and not eicosapentaenoic acid (EPA) lowered ambulatory blood pressure in overweight men. They subsequently reported from the same cohort, that DHA significantly enhanced dilatory responses to sodium nitroprusside and attenuated constrictor responses to norepinephrine (Mori et al. 2000). In studies of rats with increased blood pressure due to renal artery stenosis, the maximum blood pressure was lower in the group fed a diet enriched with DHA (Rousseau et al. 2001).

How DHA may induce a lowering of blood pressure is uncertain. Engler and Engler (2002) investigated the vasorelaxant properties of DHA in spontaneously hypertensive rats. Their results indicated that DHA's vasorelaxant actions are independent of endothelium-derived nitric oxide but may be related to modulation of intracellular calcium release and L-type calcium channels in vascular smooth muscle cells (McLauren Dorrance et al. 2000). Whether DHA has an effect on steroid and eicosanoid metabolism has also been investigated in spontaneously hypertensive rats (Engler et al. 1999a). DHA fed rats had significantly lower blood pressures than controls and the adrenal glomerulosa cells from DHA fed rats produced less aldosterone *in vitro* in response to angiotensin II, adrenocorticotrophic hormone (ACTH) or potassium.

Data relating n-6 fatty acids to effects on blood pressure are more limited. Langley-Evans and colleagues showed that systolic blood pressure of weanling male rats was inversely related to linoleic acid intake (Langley-Evans et al. 1996). Further work has indicated that 18:3 n-6 has greater hypotensive effects than its parent linoleic acid. It is postulated that the effectiveness of 18:3 n-6 may result from it being a substrate for the synthesis of a post-delta 6-desaturation metabolite that can be directly converted to blood pressure regulating eicosanoids in the kidney (Huang et al. 1994).

4 Conclusions

Data from this study support the concept of early nutritional intervention being associated with health benefits in later life. Whether the influence of LCPUFAs on blood pressure would have been more marked with a longer period of supplementation is uncertain and requires further investigation, however, an experimental rat study demonstrated that n-3 deficiency limited to the perinatal period was associated with raised blood pressure in later life, and this was not prevented by subsequent fatty acid repletion (Weisinger et al. 2001).

References

Cunnane SC, Francescutti V, Brenna JT, Crawford MA (2000). Breast-fed infants achieve a higher rate of brain and whole body docosahexaenoate accumulation than formula-fed infants not consuming dietary docosahexaenoate. *Lipids* **35**: 105–111.

Damsgaard CT, Schack-Nielsen L, Michaelsen KF, Fruekilde M-B, Hels O, Lauritzen L (2006). Fish oil affects blood pressure and the plasma lipid profile in healthy Danish infants. *J Nutr* **136**: 94–99.

Engler MB, Engler MM (2002). Docosahexaenoic acid-induced vasorelaxation in hypertensive rats: mechanisms of action. *Biol Res Nurs* **2**(2): 85–95.

Engler MM, Engler MB, Goodfriend TL, Ball DL, Yu Z, Su P, Kroetz DL (1999a). Docosahexaenoic acid is an antihypertensive nutrient that affects aldosterone production in SHR. *Proc Soc Exp Biol Med* **221**: 32–38.

Engler MM, Engler MB, Kroetz DL, Boswell KD, Neeley N, Krassner SM (1999b). The effects of a diet rich in docosahexaenoic acid on organ and vascular fatty acid composition in spontaneously hypertensive rats. *Prostaglandins Leukot Essent Fatty Acids* **61**: 289–295.

Forsyth JS, Varma S, Colvin M (1999). A randomised controlled study of the effect of long chain polyunsaturated fatty acid supplementation on stool hardness during formula feeding. *Arch Dis Child* **81**: 253–256.

Forsyth JS, Willatts P, Agostoni C, Bissenden J, Casaer P, Boehm G (2003). Long chain polyunsaturated fatty acid supplementation in infant formula and blood pressure in later childhood: follow up of cohort of children in Dundee infant feeding study. *BMJ* **326**: 953–957.

Huang YS, Cantrill RC, DeMarco A, Campbell L, Lin X, Horrobin DF, Mills DE (1994). Differences in the metabolism of 18:2 n-6 and 18:3 n-6 by the liver and kidney mat explain the anti-hypertensive effect of 18:3 n-6. *Biochem Med Metab Biol* **51**: 27–34.

Koletzko B, Agostoni C, Carlson SE, Clandinin T, Hornstra G, Neuringer M, Uauy R, Yamashiro Y, Willatts P (2001). Long chain polyunsaturated fatty acids (LC-PUFA) and perinatal development. *Acta Paediatr* **90**: 460–464.

Langley-Evans SC, Clamp AG, Grimble RF, Jackson AA (1996). Influence of dietary fats upon systolic blood pressure in the rat. *Int J Food Sci Nutr* **47**: 417–425.

Larnkjaer A, Christensen JH, Michaelson KF, Lauritzen L (2006). Maternal fish oil supplementation during lactation does not affect blood pressure, pulse wave velocity, or heart rate variability in 2.5y old children. *J Nutr* **136**: 1539–1544.

Makrides M, Neumann MA, Simmer K, Gibson RA (2000). A critical appraisal of the role of dietary long-chain polyunsaturated fatty acids on neural indices of term infants: a randomised, controlled trial. *Pediatrics* **105**: 32–38.

McLauren Dorrance A, Graham D, Dominiczak A, Fraser R (2000). Inhibition of nitric oxide synthesis increases erythrocyte membrane fluidity and unsaturated fatty acid content. *Am J Hypertens* **13**: 1194–1202.

Mori TA, Beilin LJ (2001). Long-chain omega 3 fatty acids, blood lipids and cardiovascular risk reduction. *Curr Opin Lipidol* **12**: 11–17.

Mori TA, Bao DQ, Burke V, Puddey IB, Beilin LJ (1999). Docosahexaenoic acid but not eicosapentaenoic acid lowers ambulatory blood pressure and heart rate in humans. *Hypertension* **34**: 253–260.

Mori TA, Watts GF, Burke V, Hilme E, Puddey IB, Beilin LJ (2000). Differential effects of eicosapentaenoic acid on vascular reactivity of the forearm microcirculation in hyperlipaemic, overweight men. *Circulation* **102**: 1264–1269.

Rousseau D, Helies-Toussaint C, Raederstorff D, Moreau Grynberg A (2001). Dietary n-3 polyunsaturated fatty acids affect the development of renovascular hypertension in rats. *Mol Cell Biochem* **225**: 109–119.

Singhal A, Cole TJ, Lucas A (2001). Early nutrition in preterm infants and later blood pressure: two cohorts after randomised trials. *Lancet* **357**: 413–419.

Taittonen L, Nuutinen M, Turtinen J, Uhari M (1996). Prenatal and postnatal factors in predicting later blood pressure among children: cardiovascular risk in young Finns. *Pediatr Res* **40**: 627–632.

Ulbak J, Lauritzen L, Hansen H, Michaelsen KF (2004). Diet and blood pressure in 2.5y old Danish children. *Am J Clin Nutr* **79**: 1095–1102.

Weisinger HS, Armitage JA, Sinclair AJ, Vingrys AJ, Burns PL, Weisinger RS (2001). Perinatal omega-3 fatty acid deficiency affects blood pressure in later life. *Nat Med* **7**: 258–259.

Willatts P, Forsyth JS, DiModugno MK, Varma S, Colvin M (1998). Effect of long-chain polyunsaturated fatty acids in infant formula on problem solving at 10 months. *Lancet* **352**: 688–691.

Wilson AC, Forsyth JS, Greene SA, Irvine L, Hau C, Howie PW (1998). Relation of infant diet to childhood health: seven year follow up of cohort in Dundee infant feeding study. *BMJ* **316**: 21–25.

Effects of Supplementing LCPUFA to the Diet of Pregnant Women: Data from RCT

Tamás Decsi

Abstract Randomised controlled trials (RCTs) investigating the effect of n-3 long-chain polyunsaturated fatty acid (LCPUFA) supplementation on pregnancy outcomes were recently systematically reviewed for both low-risk (uncomplicated) and high-risk pregnancies. The duration of pregnancy was found to be significantly enhanced by n-3 LCPUFA supplementation in low-risk (two systematic reviews, weighted mean difference: 2.55 and 1.57 days, 95% CI: 1.13–4.07 and 0.35–2.78 days), but not in high-risk pregnancies. The relative risk of giving birth before the 34th week of gestation was found to be reduced by n-3 LCPUFA supplementation both in low-risk (0.69, 95% CI: 0.49–0.99) and in high-risk (0.39, 95% CI: 0.19–0.84) pregnancies. Recent evidence indicates that enhancement of maternal intake of n-3 LCPUFA prolongs the duration of gestation in low-risk pregnancies and may contribute to the prevention of early preterm birth in both low-risk and high-risk pregnancies.

Keywords Docosahexaenoic acid • long-chain polyunsaturated fatty acid • pregnancy

Abbreviations DHA: docosahexaenoic acid (C22:6n-3); LCPUFA: long-chain polyunsaturated fatty acid; RCT: randomised controlled trial; RR: relative risk; SR: systematic review

1 Introduction

Long-chain polyunsaturated fatty acids (LCPUFAs) have gained increasing importance in infant nutrition during the last decades. Systematic reviews (SRs) summarizing the data of randomised controlled trials (RCTs) on the effect of the supplementation

T. Decsi
Department of Paediatrics, University of Pécs, Pécs, Hungary
tamas.decsi@aok.pte.hu

of the principal n-3 LCPUFA, docosahexaenoic acid (DHA, C22:6n-3) to full-term infants showed benefit of the supplementation both on the maturation of visual functions (Decsi and Koletzko 2000; Uauy et al. 2003) and on some cognitive domains of development (Cohen et al. 2005). However, a review of the Cochrane Collaboration concluded that there was little evidence to support the benefit of LCPUFA supplementation to full-term infants (Simmer 2001). The discrepancy between observations in apparently similar studies may originate, at least in part, from the different LCPUFA status of the infants at birth. Here we discuss data reported in recent RCTs and SRs on the effect of supplementing LCPUFAs to the diet of expectant women.

2 Effect of n-3 LCPUFA Supplementation to the Diet of Expectant Women on Maternal and Fetal Pregnancy Outcomes

RCTs investigating the effect of n-3 LCPUFA supplementation on pregnancy outcomes were recently systematically reviewed for both uncomplicated (low-risk) (Makrides et al. 2006; Szajewska et al. 2006) and high-risk pregnancies (Horvath et al. 2007). The two SRs evaluating n-3 LCPUFA supplementation in uncomplicated (low-risk) pregnancies each summarised data obtained in six RCTs. However, only two of the six trials included by Makrides et al. (2006) were also included among the six RCTs considered by Szajewska et al. (2006).

In spite of the considerable dissimilarity of the databases of the two SRs (Makrides et al. 2006; Szajewska et al. 2006), similar effects of n-3 LCPUFA supplementation on basic parameters of pregnancy outcomes were reported (Table 1). In both SRs, the duration of pregnancy was found to be significantly longer in expectant women receiving n-3 LCPUFA supplementation than in non-supplemented controls. However, in neither of the SRs was the longer pregnancy duration accompanied by significant reduction of the relative risk (RR) of giving birth prematurely; i.e. before the 37th week of gestation (Table 1). In contrast, the RR of early preterm birth (i.e. birth before the 34th week of gestation) was found to be significantly reduced in

Table 1 Basic parameters of pregnancy outcomes in systematic reviews on the effect of LCPUFA supplementation in uncomplicated (low-risk) pregnancies

Parameter	Makrides et al. (2006)	Szajewska et al. (2006)
Duration of pregnancy (day, WMD)	2.55 (1.13–4.07)	1.57 (0.35–2.78)
Birth before 37th week (RR)	0.92 (0.79–1.07)	0.67 (0.41–1.10)
Birth before 34th week (RR)	0.69 (0.49–0.99)	NR
Birth weight (g, WMD)	47 (1–93)	54 (−3–111)
Birth length (cm, WMD)	0.48 (0.13–0.83)	0.23 (−0.04–0.50)
Head circumference (cm, WMD)	NR	0.26 (0.02–0.49)

Data in brackets show 95% confidence intervals. NR = not reported, RR = relative risk; WMD = weighted mean difference (supplemented minus non-supplemented).

the supplemented group in the SR of Makrides et al. (2006), whereas this parameter was not reported in the SR of Szajewska et al. (2006).

It can be assumed with good reason that significant enhancement of the duration of physiological (uncomplicated, low-risk) pregnancy should be accompanied with increased values of anthropometric indices of the newborn. Indeed, significant increases in birth weight, birth length and head circumference at birth were found in infants of mothers receiving n-3 LCPUFA supplementation as compared to those receiving placebo in at least one of the two SRs (Makrides et al. 2006; Szajewska et al. 2006) (Table 1). In summary, data reported in the two SRs discussed above provide some evidence for the effect of n-3 LCPUFA supplementation to enhance the duration of uncomplicated (low-risk) pregnancies and, consequently, to increase to some extent birth weight, birth length and head circumference of the offspring.

Recently Horvath et al. (2007) systematically reviewed the effect of supplementation of women in high-risk pregnancies with LCPUFAs on pregnancy outcomes and growth measures at birth. This SR included four RCTs of good quality; however, several data on the duration of pregnancy and birth weight were reported only in two or three of the four RCTs. No difference was seen in the RR of duration of pregnancy exceeding 37 weeks (RR: 0.99, 95% CI: 0.9–1.1) in the two studies reporting RR values. In contrast, a significant difference (8.5 [1.9] days, mean [SD]) was found in the RCT that reported the duration of pregnancy in days (supplemented group: 269.2 [19.7] days, non-supplemented group: 260.7 [29.5] days). While no association of LCPUFA supplementation with risk of delivery before the 37th week of gestation was found (RR: 0.82, 95% CI: 0.60–1.12), the risk of early preterm delivery defined as birth before the 34th week of gestation was reduced (RR: 0.39, 95% CI: 0.19–0.84). Birth weight did not differ significantly between the supplemented and non-supplemented groups. In summary, SR of data on LCPUFA supplementation in high-risk pregnancies (Horvath et al. 2007) indicated partly similar effects to those reported for uncomplicated (low-risk) pregnancies (Makrides et al. 2006; Szajewska et al. 2006); however, the more limited database allows only weaker conclusions to be drawn.

3 Effect of n-3 LCPUFA Supplementation to the Diet of Expectant Women on Postnatal Development of the Offspring

Several aspects of postnatal development have been investigated in infants and children of mothers who received n-3 LCPUFA supplementation during pregnancy. We recently systematically reviewed RCTs published between December 2002 and September 2004 (Decsi and Koletzko 2005); however, limitations of space do not allow a systematic approach within the present paper. Hence, here we provide one example each of RCTs addressing the questions of the effect of maternal n-3 LCPUFA supplementation on visual development, cognitive development and on allergic sensitisation.

3.1 Retinal Development

Retinal development was assessed within the first week of life with full-field electroretinograms in full-term infants whose mothers received n-3 LCPUFA supplementation or placebo during pregnancy (Malcolm et al. 2003a). Electroretinogram implicite times, amplitudes and parameters of the stimulus–response function did not differ. However, linear regression analysis revealed significant association between the maturity of the retina and the availability of DHA at birth (Malcolm et al. 2003a). In the same study population, visual evoked potentials were recorded to flash stimuli shortly after birth and to both flash stimuli and pattern-reversal stimuli at 50 and 66 weeks post conception (Malcolm et al. 2003b). There were no differences between the supplementation groups; however, maturity of the pattern-reversal visual evoked potentials at 50 and 66 weeks post conception was significantly associated with the DHA status of the infant at birth (Malcolm et al. 2003b).

3.2 Cognitive Development

The cognitive development of children born from mothers receiving n-3 LCPUFA supplementation during pregnancy was studied by using the Kaufman Assessment Battery for Children at the age of 4 years (Helland et al. 2003). Children who were born to mothers receiving n-3 LCPUFA supplementation during pregnancy and lactation scored better in the mental processing tests when compared to children whose mothers did not receive n-3 LCPUFA supplementation. Multiple regression analysis suggested that maternal DHA intake during pregnancy was the only statistically significant variable for the children's mental processing scores at the age of 4 years (Helland et al. 2003).

3.3 Allergic Sensitisation

In the RCT of Dunstan et al. (2003), infants whose mothers received DHA supplementation were three times less likely to have a positive skin prick test to egg at 1 year of age than the infants whose mothers received placebo. The prevalence of atopic dermatitis did not differ; however, infants in the n-3 LCPUFA group had also significantly less severe symptoms of atopic dermatitis than infants in the control group.

4 Conclusions

There are several ongoing RCTs (e.g. Krauss-Etschmann et al. 2007) in which expectant mothers received n-3 LCPUFA supplementation during pregnancy, and various aspects of the development of their offspring are being currently investigated in a follow-up manner. Results of these RCTs will certainly contribute to our better understanding of the role of maternal n-3 LCPUFA intakes in influencing not only pregnancy outcomes, but also of the development of the infant and child as well.

Acknowledgments The work of the author was financially supported by the European Union, Sixth Framework "Early Nutrition Programming Project" FOOD-CT-2005-007036.

References

Cohen, J.T., D.C. Bellinger, W.E. Connor, B.A. Shaywitz (2005) "A quantitative analysis of prenatal intake of n-3 polyunsaturated fatty acids and cognitive development." *Am J Prev Med* **29**:366–374.

Decsi, T. and B. Koletzko (2000) "Role of long-chain polyunsaturated fatty acids in early human neurodevelopment." *Nutr Neurosci* **3**:293–306.

Decsi, T. and B. Koletzko (2005) "N-3 fatty acids and pregnancy outcomes." *Curr Opin Clin Nutr Metab Care* **8**:161–166.

Dunstan, J.A., T.A. Mori, A. Barden, L.J. Beilin, A.L. Taylor, P.G. Holt, S.L. Prescott (2003) "Fish oil supplementation in pregnancy modifies neonatal allergen-specific immune responses and clinical outcomes in infants at high risk of atopy: a randomized, controlled trial." *J Allergy Clin Immunol* **112**:1178–1184.

Helland, I.B., L. Smith, K. Saarem, O.D. Saugstad, Drevon, C.A. (2003) "Maternal supplementation with very-long-chain n-3 fatty acids during pregnancy and lactation augments children's IQ at 4 years of age." *Pediatrics* **111**:e39–e44.

Horvath, A., B. Koletzko, H. Szajewska (2007) "Effect of supplementation of women in high-risk pregnancies with long-chain polyunsaturated fatty acids on pregnancy outcomes and growth measures at birth: a meta-analysis of randomized controlled trials." *Brit J Nutr* **10**:1–7 (Epub ahead of print).

Krauss-Etschmann, S., R. Shadid, C. Campoy, E. Hoster, H. Demmelmair, M. Jiménez, A. Gil, M. Rivero, B. Veszprémi, T. Decsi, B.V. Koletzko, Nutrition and Health Lifestyle (NUHEAL) Study Group (2007) "Effects of fish-oil and folate supplementation of pregnant women on maternal and fetal plasma concentrations of docosahexaenoic acid and eicosapentaenoic acid: a European randomized multicenter trial." *Am J Clin Nutr* **85**:1392–1400.

Makrides, M., L. Duley, S.F. Olsen (2006) "Marine oil, and other prostaglandin precursor, supplementation for pregnancy uncomplicated by pre-eclampsia or intrauterine growth restriction." *Cochrane Database Syst Rev* **CD003402**.

Malcolm, C.A., R. Hamilton, D.L. McCulloch, C. Montgomery, L.T. Weaver (2003a) "Scotopic electroretinogram in term infants born of mothers supplemented with docosahexaenoic acid during pregnancy." *Invest Ophthalmol Vis Sci* **44**:3685–3691.

Malcolm, C.A., D.L. McCulloch, C. Montgomery, A. Shepherd, L.T. Weaver (2003b) "Maternal docosahexaenoic acid supplementation during pregnancy and visual evoked potential development in term infants: a double blind, prospective, randomised trial." *Arch Dis Child Fetal Neonatal Ed* **88**:F383–F390.

Simmer, K (2001) "Longchain polyunsaturated fatty acid supplementation in infants born at term." *Cochrane Database Syst Rev* **CD000376**.

Szajewska, H., A. Horvath, B. Koletzko (2006) "Effect of n-3 long-chain polyunsaturated fatty acid supplementation of women with low-risk pregnancies on pregnancy outcomes and growth measures at birth: a meta-analysis of randomized controlled trials" *Am J Clin Nutr* **83**:1337–1344.

Uauy, R., D.R. Hoffman, P. Mena, A. Llanos, E.E. Birch (2003) "Term infant studies of DHA and ARA supplementation on neurodevelopment: results of randomized controlled trials." *J Pediatr* **143**:S17–S25.

The Early Origins of Later Obesity: Pathways and Mechanisms

I. Caroline McMillen, Leewen Rattanatray, Jaime A. Duffield, Janna L. Morrison, Severence M. MacLaughlin, Sheridan Gentili, and Beverley S. Muhlhausler

Abstract Excess bodyweight is the sixth most important risk factor contributing to the overall burden of disease worldwide. In excess of a billion adults and 10% of all children are now classified as overweight or obese. The main adverse consequences of obesity are the metabolic syndrome, cardiovascular disease and type 2 diabetes and a diminished average life expectancy. It has been argued that the complex pathological processes underlying obesity reflect environmental and genetic interactions, and individuals from disadvantaged communities seem to have greater risks than more affluent individuals partly because of fetal and postnatal programming interactions. Abundant evidence indicates that the obesity epidemic reflects progressive secular and age-related decreases in physical activity, together with passive over-consumption of energy dense foods despite neurobiological processes designed to regulate energy balance. The difficulty in treating obesity, however, highlights the deficits in our current understanding of the pathophysiology which underlies the initiation and chronic nature of this disorder. Large population based studies in Europe and North America in healthy women and in women with gestational diabetes have demonstrated that there are clear relationships between maternal and fetal nutrient supply, fetal growth patterns and the subsequent risk of obesity and glucose intolerance in childhood and adult life. In this review we discuss the impact of fetal nutrition on the biology of the developing adipocyte and brain and the growing evidence base supporting an intergenerational cycle of obesity.

Keywords Appetite • fetus • leptin • obesity • programming

I.C. McMillen(✉), L. Rattanatray, J.A. Duffield, J.L. Morrison, S.M. MacLaughlin, S. Gentili, and B.S. Muhlhausler
Early Origins of Adult Health Research Group, Sansom Research Institute,
University of South Australia, Adelaide, SA 5005, Australia
caroline.mcmillen@unisa.edu.au

L. Rattanatray and J.A. Duffield
Discipline of Physiology, School of Molecular and Biomedical Sciences,
University of Adelaide, Adelaide SA 5000, Australia

B. Koletzko et al. (eds.), *Early Nutrition Programming and Health Outcomes in Later Life: Obesity and Beyond*,

Abbreviations AgRP: agouti-related protein; ARC: arcuate nucleus; BMI: body mass index; CART: cocaine- and amphetamine-regulated transcript; DMN: dorsomedial nucleus; G3PDH: glycerol 3 phosphate dehydrogenase; LPL: lipoprotein lipase; NPY: neuropeptide Y; OB-RB: leptin receptor; PVN: paraventricular nucleus; POMC: pro-opiomelanocortin; PPAR: peroxisomal proliferator-activated receptors; RXR: retinoid X receptor

1 Introduction

1.1 Birth Weight and Later Obesity

Currently more than half of all adults in the US, UK and Australia are either overweight with a body mass index (BMI) over 25 kg/m^2 or are obese with a BMI over 30 kg/m^2 and there are increasing rates of overweight and obesity in all age groups including women of reproductive age (Flegal et al. 2002; LaCoursiere et al. 2005; Ogden et al. 2006). A recent study by La Coursiere et al. (2005) found that the incidence of women being overweight or obese at the start of pregnancy increased from 25% to 35% between 1991 and 2001, and that the incidence of maternal obesity at delivery rose from 29% to 39% across the same period. A high maternal BMI increases the risk of developing hypertension, preeclampsia and gestational diabetes mellitus and of giving birth to a macrosomic infant (birth weight > 4,000 g) (Galtier-Dereure et al. 2000; Jensen et al. 2003). It has been proposed that high nutritional consumption or body fat mass during pregnancy is associated with induction of a degree of maternal insulin resistance, an increased fetal nutrient supply, fetal overgrowth and infant fatness (Catalano et al. 2003). Whilst it is not unexpected that the maternal nutritional and hormonal environment would determine fetal nutrient supply and infant body composition, it appears that the effects of the nutritional environment experienced *in utero* persist beyond fetal life. An extensive series of studies has reported that there is a J or U shaped relationship between birth weight and adult fat mass, with a higher prevalence of adult obesity occurring in individuals with birth weights which were at either the low or high end of the birth weight distribution (Curhan et al. 1996a, b; Fall et al. 1995; Maffeis et al. 1994; Parsons et al. 2001).

A study in a large British cohort (n = 10,683) found that the low birth weight babies who were most vulnerable to developing obesity were light and thin at birth and then experienced a period of rapid growth in the first 7 years of life (Parsons et al. 2001). In contrast, babies who were in the heaviest quintile of birth weight, tended to have a high BMI in adult life independent of their rate of childhood growth and this relationship was largely accounted for by maternal weight and was independent of maternal height, paternal height, socio-economic status or smoking habits. Thus heavier mothers have heavier babies and these babies have a high BMI in adult life. A recent Danish study of 300,000 children born between 1936 and 1983 also reported a remarkably stable association between having a birth weight greater than 4,000 g and being overweight at 6–13 years of age (Rugholm et al. 2005).

1.2 Perinatal Nutrition and Later Obesity

In mothers with gestational diabetes, maternal and fetal blood glucose concentrations are higher, resulting in fetal hyperinsulinaemia, fetal overgrowth and an increased fetal adiposity and hyperleptinaemia. Interestingly in pregnancies complicated by gestational diabetes or even mildly impaired glucose tolerance, the offspring are at risk of developing obesity and glucose intolerance in later life (Oken and Gillman 2003; Silverman et al. 1991). The period during which exposure to increased energy supply may have a longer term impact on the nutritional environment may extend beyond the prenatal period into infancy and early childhood. Rapid weight gain during the first weeks or months of life has been shown to be associated with an increased risk of being overweight or obese in childhood and in early adult life (Ekelund et al. 2006; Stettler et al. 2002, 2003, 2005).

In a large, prospective contemporary cohort study, dietary energy intake in formula- or mixed-fed infants at as early as 4 months of age was positively related to early childhood weight gain and subsequent body weight and BMI up to 5 years of age (Ong et al. 2006). In a separate study, it was also reported that each 100 g increase in absolute weight gain during the first week of infancy was associated

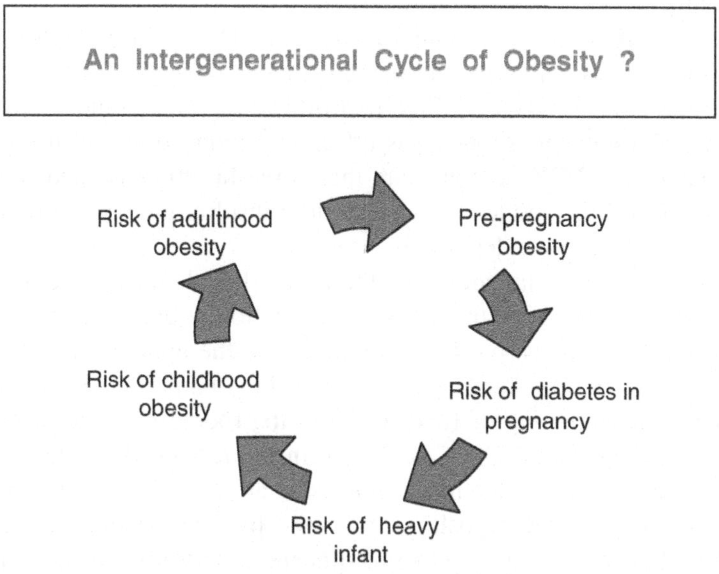

Fig. 1 The intergenerational cycle of obesity

with a 28% increase in the risk of becoming an overweight adult (Stettler et al. 2005). The authors of this study concluded that if the causality was confirmed, that 'new strategies based on a life course approach' using short interventions in early infancy may be useful to prevent obesity and related metabolic health risk factors. Thus it has been proposed that there may be an intergenerational cycle of obesity based on the associations between exposure to an increased energy supply during the perinatal period and being overweight or obese in childhood and later life (Fig. 1). Whilst the mechanisms underlying these associations are unknown, the two primary targets for the perinatal programming of obesity are the developing fat cell, the adipocyte, and the neuroendocrine network which regulates appetite and energy balance in adult life.

2 Maternal Overnutrition and Postnatal Adiposity: Experimental Animal Studies

In the adult, appetite and energy balance homeostasis are primarily regulated by a complex neuronal circuitry located within the hypothalamus which receives nutrient, hormonal and neural signals from a range of sources including fat cells, the pancreas, the gastrointestinal tract and other brain regions. A range of neuropeptides including the orexigenic neuropeptides, neuropeptide Y (NPY) and agouti-related protein (AgRP), and the anorexigenic neuropeptides, pro-opiomelanocortin (POMC) and cocaine- and amphetamine-regulated transcript (CART), are expressed within the hypothalamus and together act in synchrony to regulate energy balance. NPY is a 36 amino acid neuropeptide which markedly stimulates appetite and is predominantly localised in the arcuate nucleus of the hypothalamus with low levels of expression within the dorsomedial nucleus (DMN). NPY neurones project to hypothalamic regions which play important roles in energy balance including the paraventricular nucleus (PVN), DMN, perifornical region and the lateral hypothalamic area. The blood brain barrier is effectively reduced within the area of the arcuate nucleus and NPY neurones are therefore able to sense and respond to a range of peripheral metabolic signals including insulin, glucose, ghrelin, and the adipocyte derived hormone, leptin.

A series of experimental studies in the rodent has demonstrated that glucose, insulin or leptin derived from the maternal circulation or present in her breast milk exert a dominant influence on the development of the appetite regulatory neural network and that the immediate postnatal period is of particular importance for the long-term programming of food intake in the rodent (Davidowa et al. 2003; Davidowa and Plagemann 2000a, b, 2001). In the rodent, the induction of mild gestational diabetes or a reduction in litter size are associated with an increased early weight gain and fat deposition, followed by hyperphagia, obesity, hyperleptinaemia, hyperglycaemia, hyperinsulinaemia and insulin resistance. The nature of the maternal metabolic and hormonal signals and the critical windows during which programming of appetite may occur in the litter-bearing, altricial rodent are likely to be different, however, from those in non-litter-bearing, precocial species such as the sheep in which development of the major fat depots and of hypothalamic neuropeptide expression occur before birth (Muhlhausler et al. 2004, 2005).

We have developed a model of maternal 'overnutrition' in which the pregnant ewe is overfed during the last month of pregnancy until delivery and we have demonstrated that there is development of an increased mass of subcutaneous fat in the lambs of overnourished ewes by as early as 30 days of age (Muhlhausler et al. 2006). In these studies increasing maternal nutrition by ~40% in late gestation significantly increased lamb milk intake and plasma glucose concentrations the first 30 days of life. The relative mass of subcutaneous adipose tissue at 30 days was also greater in lambs of well fed ewes (40.0 ± 3.9 g/kg vs. 22.1 ± 3.5 g/kg, $P < 0.05$). In order to determine the mechanisms which underlie the increase in subcutaneous adiposity, we have measured the effect of the increased maternal nutrition on the expression of adipogenic and lipogenic genes in perirenal fat, the major fat depot present before birth and in perirenal and subcutaneous fat at 30 days.

2.1 *Maternal Nutrition and Adipogenesis in Fetal Visceral Adipose Tissue*

The peroxisomal proliferator-activated receptors (PPARs) are members of the nuclear hormone receptor superfamily that bind to specific DNA response elements as heterodimers with the retinoid X receptor (RXR). The *PPARγ* gene produces two proteins, PPARγ1 and the adipose-specific PPARγ2. Expression of PPARγ is highest in adipose tissue, where it regulates the transcriptional cascade underlying adipogenesis (Semple et al. 2006). The ligand-binding pocket of PPARγ allows unsaturated fatty acids, oxidized lipid species, eicosanoids, and prostaglandins to activate the receptor and transduce nutritional signals into metabolic responses. Activation of PPARγ by specific ligands such as the thiazolidinediones (TZDs) increases the expression of genes involved in the storage of triglycerides within adipose cells, including lipoprotein lipase (LPL) and glycerol 3 phosphate dehydrogenase G3PDH and increases the expression of the insulin sensitising hormone, adiponectin, within adipose tissue.

We have recently carried out the first study to investigate the impact of maternal overnutrition on expression of PPARγ mRNA expression in visceral adipose tissue before birth. Maternal overnutrition imposed between 115–141 days gestation (term = 150 ± 3 days gestation) resulted in a significant increase in circulating fetal glucose and insulin concentrations (Muhlhausler et al. 2007). Whilst the relative mass of fetal perirenal fat was not increased in the overnourished group by 141 days gestation, the expression of PPARγ, LPL, adiponectin and leptin mRNA

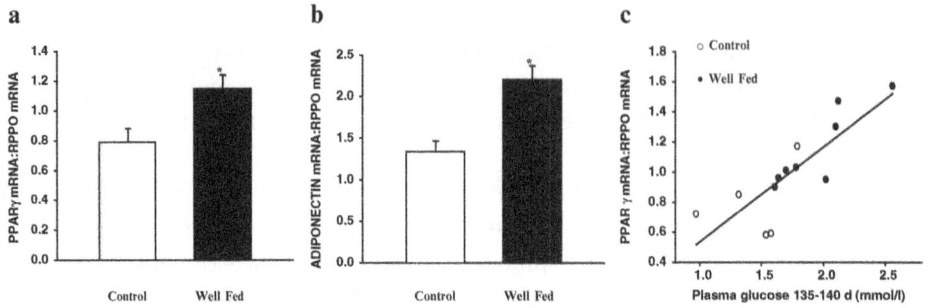

Fig. 2 Maternal overnutrition in late gestation resulted in an increase in the expression of PPARγ and Adiponectin mRNA in fetal adipose tissue (**a** and **b**). There was a direct relationship between PPARγ expression and mean plasma glucose concentrations when data from all fetuses were combined (**c**) (Reproduced with permission from Muhlhausler et al. 2007)

in fetal perirenal fat was each significantly higher in those from the overnourished ewes at this gestational age (see Fig. 2). Furthermore, there were significant relationships between the level of PPARγ mRNA expression in fetal fat and the mean fetal plasma glucose or insulin concentrations during late gestation (Fig. 2). The expression of LPL, G3PDH and adiponectin, but not leptin, were each significantly positively related to PPARγ mRNA expression in fetal fat. One possibility is therefore that an increase in fetal nutrition increases the expression and activation of the adipogenic gene, PPARγ, in perirenal adipose tissue and that there is then subsequent endocrine signalling, between the perirenal adipocytes which develop in fetal life, and the subcutaneous adipocytes which develop predominantly around the time of birth.

2.2 *Maternal Nutrition and the Programming of the Central Regulation of Energy Balance*

We have previously reported that genes for the appetite regulating neuropeptides NPY, AgRP, POMC and CART are each highly expressed in the ventromedial portion of the arcuate nucleus (ARC) of the fetal sheep hypothalamus by 110 days gestation, which is consistent with their pattern of expression in the adult sheep hypothalamus (Muhlhausler et al. 2004). Furthermore, and in contrast to the rodent, NPY projections are also present in the fetal paraventricular nucleus (PVN) during late gestation (Warnes et al. 1998). Messenger RNA for the long form of the leptin receptor (OB-Rb) is also expressed in both the ARC and ventromedial nucleus of the fetal sheep hypothalamus (Muhlhausler et al. 2004). In our recently published studies in the fetus and lamb of the overnourished ewes we have also used *in situ* hybridisation to investigate the impact of maternal nutrition on the expression of the neuropeptides in the hypothalamic arcuate nucleus which either act to stimulate appetite in postnatal life (NPY and AGRP) or inhibit it (CART and POMC) (Muhlhausler et al. 2006). We found that there was no difference in the expression of either NPY or AgRP mRNA between the control and well fed groups, in either the fetal or lamb hypothalamus, however we found that in the lamb, but not in the fetus, NPY and AgRP mRNA expressions were each inversely related to adiposity (total fat: NPY = –0.005 total fat + 0.89 $P < 0.05$, n = 16; AgRP = –0.007 total fat + 0.95 $P < 0.01$, n = 17). These findings suggest that signals of current nutritional status or lamb fat stores, rather than nutrition during the prenatal period, may be the more important determinants of NPY and AgRP expression in early postnatal life.

Exposure to increased maternal nutrition in late pregnancy also resulted in a change in the relationship between expression of CART mRNA in the hypothalamic arcuate nucleus and the relative body fat mass. Although CART mRNA expression was positively correlated with relative adiposity and plasma leptin concentrations in control lambs, these relationships were not present in lambs of well-fed ewes (Fig. 3). It would therefore appear that the sensitivity of the CART-expressing neurons in the ARC to signals of increased nutrient supply and body fat mass may be reduced in lambs exposed to an increased supply of nutrients before birth, which would have important implications for the subsequent regulation of energy balance homeostasis. Furthermore in lambs of well fed ewes, but not their control counterparts, there was a significant inverse relationship between the hypothalamic expression of OBRb mRNA in the arcuate nucleus and total relative fat mass at 30 days (Muhlhausler et al. 2006) (Fig. 3). Thus, in lambs of

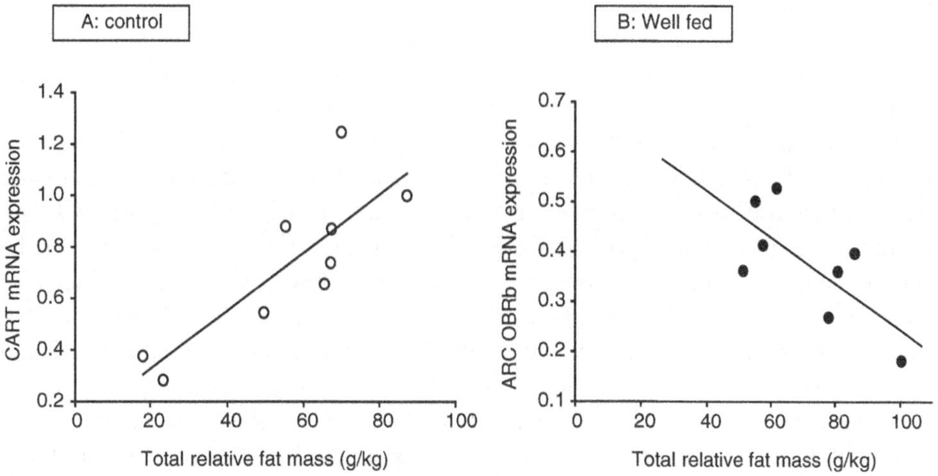

Fig. 3 There was a significant positive relationship between CART mRNA expression and total relative fat mass in the Control group but not Well Fed group (**A**). There was an inverse relationship between OBRb mRNA expression in the arcuate nucleus (ARC) and total relative fat mass in the Well Fed group (**B**) (Reproduced with permission from Muhlhausler et al. 2006)

well fed ewes, the expression of OBRb was down regulated as fat mass increased, which suggests that the sensitivity of these lambs to circulating leptin decreased with increasing adiposity. It has been shown that the density of neuronal connections between hypothalamic nuclei, and therefore the subsequent function of the neural network regulating appetite, is strongly influenced by the availability of leptin during hypothalamic development (Bouret et al. 2004). One possibility, therefore, is that the differential regulation of CART in the control and well-fed groups is a consequence of programmed changes to the hypothalamic architecture. Thus metabolic or hormonal signals could act during the perinatal period to alter the structural and functional properties of the central neural network that regulates energy balance during adult life.

3 Summary

A growing body of evidence from both epidemiological and experimental animal studies has clearly demonstrated that exposure to an elevated or excessive nutrient supply before birth is associated with an increased risk of obesity and associated metabolic disorders in later life. The global epidemic of obesity is a phenomena which demands a solution and this solution in turn demands an increased understanding of the underlying etiology of obesity, particular those factors which can be realistically modified. Whilst lifestyle and environmental factors clearly play a part – there is increasing evidence that the origins of obesity may be very early in life – and may be related strongly to the prenatal and perinatal nutritional experience of an individual.

We have previously reported in the sheep – an animal model in which the systems which regulate fat deposition and appetite develop before birth, as in the human – that exposure to an increased nutrient supply before birth is associated with an increase (upregulation) of the expression of genes which regulate adipogenesis (PPARγ) and lipogenesis (LPL) in adipose tissue before birth, and is associated with an increase in subcutaneous fat mass as early as 1 month of postnatal age. Furthermore, in lambs of well fed ewes, expression of the leptin receptor in the central neural network decreased with increasing adiposity, and the capacity to increase expression of the central appetite-inhibiting neuropeptide, CART, was lost. Based on these findings, we speculate that the early upregulation of adipogenic and lipogenic genes before birth is associated with a greater lipogenic capacity within these adipocytes as the individual emerges into an extrauterine environment, which results in an increased fat deposition in early postnatal life. We suggest that these findings present an argument for the primacy of changes within the adipose tissue – i.e. the establishment of an increased fat mass through a change in the structural and functional properties of the adipocyte, which leads to a greater potential for the accumulation of adipose tissue after birth, suppresses expression of the leptin receptor at central sites and propagates a phenotype of obesity and leptin resistance throughout the life-course (see Fig. 4).

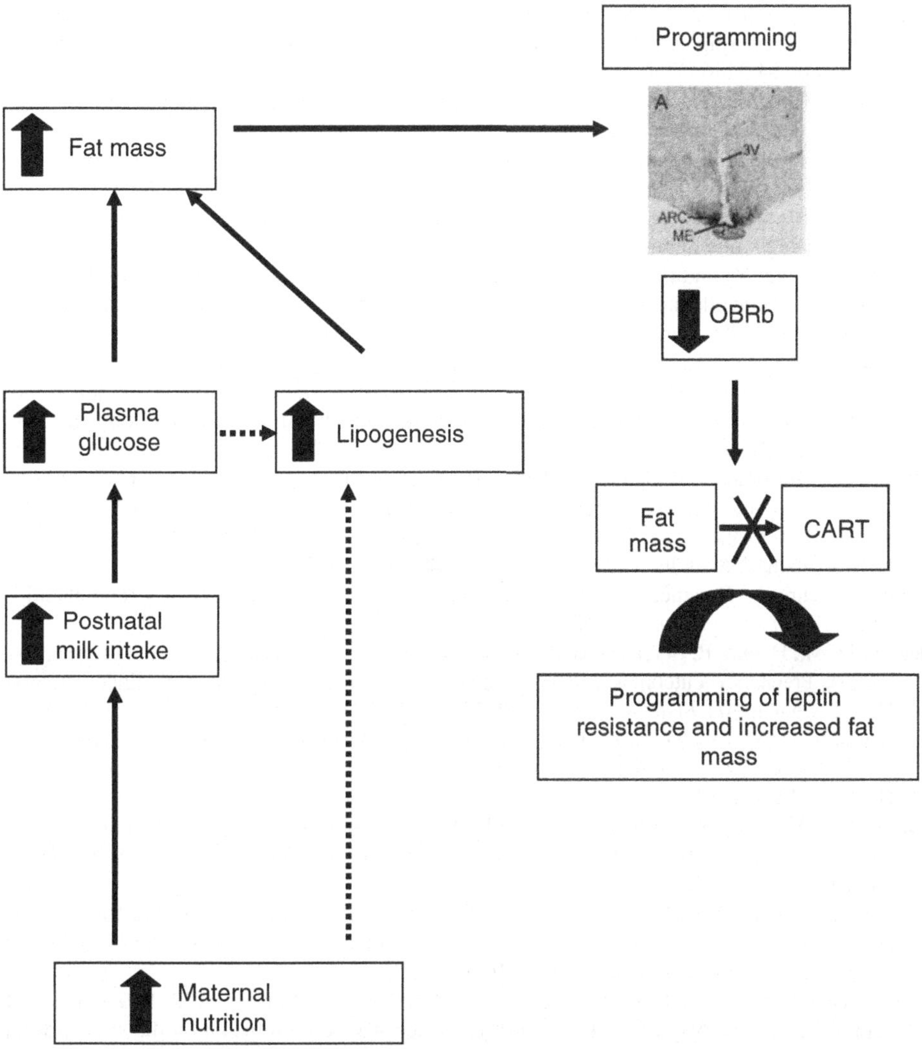

Fig. 4 Summary of the potential mechanisms for the programming of obesity in response to an increased nutrient supply before birth

References

Bouret, S. G., Draper, S. J., and Simerly, R. B. (2004). Trophic action of leptin on hypothalamic neurons that regulate feeding. *Science* **304**:108–110.

Catalano, P. M., Kirwan, J. P., Haugel-de Mouzon, S., and King, J. (2003). Gestational diabetes and insulin resistance: role in short- and long-term implications for mother and fetus. *J Nutr* **133**:1674S–1683S.

Curhan, G. C., Chertow, G. M., Willett, W. C., Spiegelman, D., Colditz, G. A., Manson, J. E., Speizer, F. E., and Stampfer, M. J. (1996a). Birth weight and adult hypertension and obesity in women. *Circulation* **94**:1310–1315.

Curhan, G. C., Willett, W. C., Rimm, E. B., Spiegelman, D., Ascherio, A. L., and Stampfer, M. J. (1996b). Birth weight and adult hypertension, diabetes mellitus, and obesity in US men. *Circulation* **94**:3246–3250.

Davidowa, H. and Plagemann, A. (2000a). Decreased inhibition by leptin of hypothalamic arcuate neurons in neonatally overfed young rats. *Neuroreport* **11**:2795–2798.

Davidowa, H. and Plagemann, A. (2000b). Different responses of ventromedial hypothalamic neurons to leptin in normal and early postnatally overfed rats. *Neurosci Lett* **293**:21–24.

Davidowa, H. and Plagemann, A. (2001). Inhibition by insulin of hypothalamic VMN neurons in rats overweight due to postnatal overfeeding. *Neuroreport* **12**:3201–3204.

Davidowa, H., Li, Y., and Plagemann, A. (2003). Altered responses to orexigenic (AGRP, MCH) and anorexigenic (alpha-MSH, CART) neuropeptides of paraventricular hypothalamic neurons in early postnatally overfed rats. *Eur J Neurosci* **18**:613–621.

Ekelund, U., Ong, K., Linne, Y., Neovius, M., Brage, S., Dunger, D. B., Wareham, N. J., and Rossner, S. (2006). Upward weight percentile crossing in infancy and early childhood independently predicts fat mass in young adults: the Stockholm Weight Development Study (SWEDES). *Am J Clin Nutr* **83**:324–330.

Fall, C. H., Osmond, C., Barker, D. J., Clark, P. M., Hales, C. N., Stirling, Y., and Meade, T. W. (1995). Fetal and infant growth and cardiovascular risk factors in women. *BMJ* **310**:428–432.

Flegal, K. M., Carroll, M. D., Ogden, C. L., and Johnson, C. L. (2002). Prevalence and trends in obesity among US adults, 1999–2000. *JAMA* **288**:1723–1727.

Galtier-Dereure, F., Boegner, C., and Bringer, J. (2000). Obesity and pregnancy: complications and cost. *Am J Clin Nutr* **71**:1242S–1248S.

Jensen, D. M., Damm, P., Sorensen, B., Molsted-Pedersen, L., Westergaard, J. G., and Ovesen, P.-H. (2003). Pregnancy outcomes and prepregnancy body mass index is 2459 glucose-tolerant Danish women. *Am J Obstet Gynecol* **189**:239–244.

LaCoursiere, D. Y., Bloebaum, L., Douncan, J. D., and Varner, M. W. (2005). Population-based trends and correlates of maternal overweight and obesity, Utah 1991–2001. *Am J Obstet Gynecol* **192**:832–839.

Maffeis, C., Micciolo, R., Must, A., Zaffanello, M., and Pineli, L. (1994). Parental and perinatal factors associated with childhood obesity in north-east Italy. *Int J Obes Relat Metab Disord* **18**:301–305.

Muhlhausler, B. S., McMillen, I. C., Rouzaud, G., Findlay, P. A., Marrocco, E. M., Rhind, S. M., and Adam, C. L. (2004). Appetite regulatory neuropeptides are expressed in the sheep hypothalamus before birth. *J Neuroendocrinol* **16**:502–507.

Muhlhausler, B. S., Adam, C. L., Marrocco, E. M., Findlay, P. A., Roberts, C. T., McFarlane, J. R., Kauter, K. G., and McMillen, I. C. (2005). Impact of glucose infusion on the structural and functional characteristics of adipose tissue and on hypothalamic gene expression for appetite regulatory neuropeptides in the sheep fetus during late gestation. *J Physiol* **565**:185–195.

Muhlhausler, B. S., Adam, C. L., Findlay, P. A., Duffield, J. A., and McMillen, I. C. (2006). Increased maternal nutrition alters development of the appetite-regulating network in the brain. *FASEB J* **20**:1257–1259.

Muhlhausler, B. S., Duffield, J. A., and McMillen, I. C. (2007). Increased maternal nutrition stimulates peroxisome proliferator activated receptor-γ (PPARγ), adiponectin and leptin mRNA expression in adipose tissue before birth. *Endocrinology* **148**:878–885.

Ogden, C. L., Carroll, M. D., Curtin, L. R., McDowell, M. A., Tabak, C. J., and Flegal, K. M. (2006). Prevalence of overweight and obesity in the United states, 1999–2004. *JAMA* **295**:1549–1555.

Oken, E. and Gillman, M. W. (2003). Fetal origins of obesity. *Obes Res* **11**:496–506.

Ong, K. K., Emmett, P. M., Noble, S., Ness, A., and Dunger, D. B. (2006). Dietary energy intake at the age of 4 months predicts postnatal weight gain and childhood body mass index. *Pediatrics* **117**:e503–e508.

Parsons, T. J., Power, C., and Manor, O. (2001). Fetal and early life growth and body mass index from birth to early adulthood in 1958 British cohort: longitudinal study. *BMJ* **323**:1331–1335.

Rugholm, S., Baker, J. L., Olsen, L. W., Schack-Nielsen, L., Bua, J., and Sorensen, T. I. A. (2005). Stability of the association between birth weight and childhood overweight during the development of the obesity epidemic. *Obes Res* **13**:2187–2194.

Semple, R. K., Chatterjee, V. K., and O'Rahilly, S. (2006). PPAR gamma and human metabolic disease. *J Clin Invest* **116**:581–589.

Silverman, B. L., Rizzo, T., Green, O. C., Cho, N. H., Winter, R. J., Ogata, E. S., Richards, G. E., and Metzger, B. E. (1991). Long-term prospective evaluation of offspring of diabetic mothers. *Diabetes* **40**:121–125.

Stettler, N., Zemel, B. S., Kumanyika, S., and Stallings, V. A. (2002). Infant weight gain and childhood overweight status in a multicenter, cohort study. *Pediatrics* **109**:194–199.

Stettler, N., Kumanyika, S. K., Katz, S. H., Zemel, B. S., and Stallings, V. A. (2003). Rapid weight gain during infancy and obesity in young adulthood in a cohort of African Americans. *Am J Clin Nutr* **77**:1374–1378.

Stettler, N., Stallings, V. A., Troxel, A. B., Zhao, J., Schinnar, R., Nelson, S. E., Ziegler, E. E., and Strom, B. L. (2005). Weight gain in the first week of life and overweight in adulthood: a cohort study of European American subjects fed infant formula. *Circulation* **111**:1897–1903.

Warnes, K. E., Morris, M. J., Symonds, M. E., Phillips, I. D., Clarke, I. J., Owens, J. A., and McMillen, I. C. (1998). Impact of gestational age, cortisol and maternal undernutrition on hypothalamic neuropeptide Y expression in the sheep fetus. *J Neuroendocrinol* **10**:51–57.

Developmental Origins of Obesity: Programming of Food Intake or Physical Activity?

David S. Gardner and Phillip Rhodes

Abstract Mans ability to capture, harness and store energy most efficiently as fat in adipose tissue has been an evolutionary success story for the majority of human existence. Only over the last 30–40 years has our remarkable metabolic efficiency been revealed as our energy balance increasingly favours storage without regular periods of depletion. Historical records show us that while the composition of our diet has changed markedly over this time, our overall energy intake has significantly reduced. The inevitable conclusion therefore is that habitual physical activity and thus energy expenditure has reduced by a greater extent. Recent studies have illustrated how the finely tuned long-term control of energy intake and of energy expenditure are both developmentally plastic and susceptible to environmentally-induced change that may persist with that individual throughout their adult life, invariably rendering them more susceptible to greater adipose tissue deposition. The central role that lean body mass has upon the 'gating' of energy sensing and the importance of regular physical activity for its potential to reduce the burden of a 'thrifty phenotype' will be briefly discussed in the present review.

Keywords Obesity • physical activity • nutrition • appetite • food intake • programming

Abbreviations ACC: acetyl-CoA carboxylase; AgRP: agouti-related peptide; GLUT4: glucose transporter 4; NEAT: non-exercise activity thermogenesis; NPY: neuropeptide Y; PPAR: peroxisome proliferator activated receptor; PPAR: gamma coactivator alpha (PGC-1α) and beta (PGC-1β); T2D: Type 2 Diabetes

---

D.S. Gardner(✉) and P. Rhodes
Centre for Reproduction and Early Life, School of Veterinary Medicine and Science, University of Nottingham, Sutton Bonington, LE12 5RD
david.gardner@nottingham.ac.uk

B. Koletzko et al. (eds.), *Early Nutrition Programming and Health Outcomes in Later Life: Obesity and Beyond*,

1 Introduction – Energy Handling in Humans

Simplistically the Universe is comprised of matter and antimatter. Matter has Mass (a relative weight) and Mass has Energy. Einstein famously described how much energy is contained within any object with mass. Energy in the universe is constant; that is, cannot be created or destroyed only transferred – the First law of Thermodynamics. Plant life first evolved the ability to harness the energy of sunlight to synthesis carbohydrate and produce adenosine triphosphate – the unit of metabolic energy. Animal life then evolved to eat the plants (herbivores), eat the herbivores (carnivores) and/or eat other carnivores and plants (omnivores). At each trophic level some of the transferred energy is lost (mainly as heat) and the absolute demand for energy to fuel metabolic processes is increased i.e. from prokaryotes to eukaryotes (fungi⇒plants⇒animals). Extant animal species have successfully evolved mechanisms to harness, transfer and store metabolic energy, with relative inefficiency an obligatory part of the process. The efficiency of metabolic energy handling is therefore an important evolutionary pressure.

In humans, using adipose tissue to store fat (as triglycerides) represents the most efficient means to 'store' energy, as it is relatively energy dense and dehydrated. In theory, adipose tissue offers a seemingly unlimited potential for energy storage, but clearly there is an asymptotic plateau in which maintenance of the excess weight becomes a significant demand in itself and reduces an individual's capacity for partitioning energy into reproduction, fertility, and body defences (immune competence) and the necessary accompanying behaviours (physical activity) that ensure continued survival. Consequently, at a species-level, man is relatively fat with a distinct sex-specific bias. Evolutionary pressures act on males to become relatively lean and large (more lean than fat mass) and females to have sufficient energy reserves and other morphometric characteristics that ensure the successful bearing of young. On a population scale therefore, men are generally taller, stronger and leaner than women. The evolutionary pressures that determined the human genotype to subsequently shape our body composition and metabolic competence (i.e. phenotype) to ensure a beneficial evolutionary advantage are, transposed into the current environment, proving too efficient; our paleolithic physiology combined with nutritional abundance without recall to physical activity, is producing an overweight and obese population. This has been described as a nutrition transition; i.e. from a hunter-gatherer society, through the agricultural and industrial revolutions that improved food security, but were often marked by periods of famine, up to a modern society characterized by freely available food and labour saving devices (Popkin 2006). On the whole and over an extended period of time, intake of energy has exceeded energy expenditure and where previously (Paleolithic era) the excess energy was regularly turned-over through physical activity, this crucial cycle has now been broken (Chakravarthy and Booth 2004). Such a process reduces metabolic flexibility and increases the rate of degeneration of tissues and organs, which combined with an aging population, is significantly increasing the burden of non-communicable disease in the world-wide population (Popkin 2006; Smyth and Heron 2006).

1.1 Obesity and the Control of Energy Balance

The tendency to store excess energy in adipose tissue as fat is multifactorial with potential aetiologies at all biological levels i.e. genetic, physiological and sociological. Although large scale associative genotyping studies have recently revealed potential genetic contributors to an individual's body fat setting or 'adipostat' (Frayling et al. 2007), clearly, obesity reflects a classic environmental*genetic interaction since if it were the case that genes entirely underpinned obesity then obesity would have been as prevalent in the past as it is today, which is not true (Keith et al. 2006). Much debate surrounds sociological aetiologies for obesity, such as societal pressures, portion sizes and marketing strategies; however, ultimately these relate to a desire to eat (appetite) balanced by sufficient activity to effectively utilise that food energy. The relative contribution ascribed to either 'overeating' or 'under-activity' is also much debated. Empirically, overall energy intake as food and drink has declined over the last 20 years (Food Standards Agency & Department of Health 2004; National Food Survey 2007) assuming dietary underreporting was as prevalent in 1974 as it is in 2007 (Bedard et al. 2004; Lissner 2002). Habitual physical activity, on the other hand, has clearly declined by a much greater extent than food intake (Kimm et al. 2005; Sothern 2004; Swinburn and Egger 2004) given the historical trends in obesity (Keith et al. 2006).

Obesity reflects a subtle loss of control of energy balance such that over time, the excess energy is stored as fat. Potential mechanisms underpinning this subtle 'loss of control' are most likely multi-faceted and widely debated, and this brief review shall concentrate on only two main areas; that of a role for the early environment in 'programming' subtle alterations to appetite and/or physical activity and the contributing role each may play in the much touted 'obesity pandemic'. While we may not be eating more energy *per se* the composition of what we now eat is markedly different to the assumed paleolithic, hunter gatherer diet on which our appetites and metabolic physiology evolved (Popkin 2006) and upon which we, even as children, were much healthier (Prynne et al. 1999). Globally, the energy density of our diet has increased: traditional African diets are ~450 kJ · 100 g^{-1} as compared to the average British diet (~670 kJ · 100 g^{-1}) or average fast-food outlet (~1,100 kJ · 100 g^{-1}) (Prentice and Jebb 2003) and have become sweeter and more refined, with more simple sugars and reduced fibre (Food Standards Agency & Department of Health 2004). Total fat intake has decreased, but saturated and artificial (e.g. *trans*) fats have increased (Food Standards Agency & Department of Health 2004). These changes largely accompany urbanisation, greater wealth, increased processed food and drink intake and decreased consumption of 'raw' foods; whole grains, fruit, vegetables (Popkin 2006). These subtle compositional changes may 'deceive' ordinary regulatory processes: for example, a 70 kg human has ~18.3 kg stored energy, of which 66.5% (12 kg), 32.8% (6 kg) and 0.7% (0.3 kg) is fat, protein and carbohydrate, respectively. This equates to 139, 200 kcal assuming oxidation of fat, protein and carbohydrate yields 9.3, 4.4 and 4.0 kcal, respectively. For total fat, daily intake relative to this 'reserve' is very small (35% of ~2,000 kcal

= 700 kcal, relative to 'reserve' of 92,568 kcal or ~0.1%) and therefore very slight changes in the fat content of food maybe more difficult to effectively sense and regulate. The modern diet is placing more emphasis on pancreatic functional capacity (increased extrinsic sugars, glycaemic index of food) and exceptional dietary regulation of intake within the context of greatly reduced need for overt physical activity. Clearly over long periods of time i.e. years–decades, such an environment facilitates a gradually increasing fat mass. Additionally, there is evidence that both may be susceptible or 'plastic' to early life programming.

2 Developmental Programming of Energy Intake and Energy Expenditure

The control of food intake through the appetite-regulatory networks in the hypothalamus has been reviewed extensively (Kalra et al. 1999) and its susceptibility through early life programming has also received much recent interest in the scientific community (Langley-Evans et al. 2005; Cripps et al. 2005; Bouret and Simerly 2006; Horvath and Bruning 2006). The mouse and rat models from which much of this work has originated has proved particularly useful in this respect due to the neonatal susceptibility of these appetite-regulatory pathways i.e. an early environment stimulus, for example being exposed to under/overnutrition when raised in large/small litters, respectively has long term consequences for food intake and food preference (Oscai and McGarr 1978; Widdowson and McCance 1975; Widdowson 1970). More recently, it has been shown that both the genetically predetermined hyperphagic and obese *ob/ob* mouse phenotype and dietary-induced obese and lethargic rat phenotype (Vickers et al. 2000) may be reversed, very simply, through neonatal exposure to leptin – the humoral 'adipostat' (Bouret and Simerly 2006; Bouret et al. 2004; Vickers et al. 2005).

The equivalent developmental period for resetting of appetite networks in larger animals such as humans and sheep occurs prenatally, during late gestation. Interestingly, an enhanced nutritional plane at this time in sheep has recently been shown to influence early appetite behaviour (Muhlhausler et al. 2006). Thus diverse and non-specific nutritional inputs can influence an immature hypothalamic appetite network to the detriment of the individual in later life i.e. they become more susceptible to poor nutritional control. A key mediator of this effect is leptin and its effects on hypothalamic reorganisation. This raises interesting questions about the role of maternal body composition, lactational performance and leptin concentration in milk (Lisboa et al. 2006; Miralles et al. 2006; Mostyn et al. 2006; Muhlhausler et al. 2006; Savino et al. 2006) – cumulatively reflected in the infant as the rate of neonatal leptin intake, which may therefore underpin many of the observed developmentally programmed effects on appetite and body composition in later life.

Interestingly, some of the main hypothalamic targets for leptin that have been shown to influence appetite control also influence energy expenditure e.g. central melanocortins (Balthasar et al. 2005). Indeed, when leptin is considered as a systemic mechanism to indicate sufficient energy 'reserves' for maintenance of growth, reproduction and immune competence then it is hardly surprising that excess energy initiates leptin-mediated hypophagia (Bouret et al. 2004) and increased energy expenditure (Mark et al. 2003) as a means to restore somatic energy balance. The central melanocortin pathways involving neurons co-expressing neuropeptide Y (NPY) and agouti-related peptide (AgRP) appear to act as the fulcrum balancing energy intake and expenditure (Balthasar et al. 2005). Indeed, alterations to these pathways either through early life experience and/or an interaction with the adult environment may produce a specific hypothalamic leptin resistance that affects both energy intake and expenditure (Enriori et al. 2007). Such a mechanism, coupled with the historical changes in food energy density and composition, may explain why excess energy is gradually stored, over time, in developmentally programmed individuals rather than sensed and regulated.

2.1 Programming of Physical Activity Level

While leptin appears to be the key humoral regulator of somatic 'energy-sensing', overall energy regulation is through variations in physical activity induced energy expenditure. On the whole energy expenditure drives energy intake rather than *vice versa.* Historically, increased physical activity would by necessity accompany periods of reduced energy intake (Chakravarthy and Booth 2004) and thus energy reserves would become depleted. In this environment any subtle changes to appetite networks were thus masked by continued feed-fast cycles. In modern life this is not happening and the continuous availability of food together with little demand for overt physical activity engenders an environment that encourages weight gain. In this environment, for potentially 'programmed' individuals i.e. those bearing hypothalamic imprints that reflect leptin resistance, excess weight gain will occur at a greater rate, clinical obesity manifests earlier and premature mortality beckons. Few studies have shown direct programming of energy expenditure. One study associated severe maternal undernutrition with both increased food intake and decreased habitual behavioural-related activity prior to maturity onset obesity (Vickers et al. 2003), first suggesting potential programming of reduced energy expenditure through reduced physical activity. Again, neonatal leptin treatment successfully reversed the deleterious effects on energy expenditure (Vickers et al. 2005). We have shown that sheep made obese through restriction of physical activity and increased availability of energy dense food (Williams et al. 2007) exhibit individual variation in physical activity level, but the rank order of activity is maintained from early into later life (Fig. 1) suggesting an individual 'activitystat'. Such a proposal is not new and was suggested earlier by Wilkin et al. based upon physical activity in school children (Wilkin et al. 2006). Indeed, non-exercise activity thermogenesis (NEAT) i.e. energy expenditure associated with ambulating but not overt physical activity has been proposed to be individually fixed early in life, and to potentially account for up to 15 kg extra fat mass per year between individuals with low or high NEAT (Levine et al. 2005). Clearly, therefore, successful balance of somatic energy transfer relies upon a threshold level of energy expenditure through physical activity. This is exemplified in studies in which overweight individuals engaged in low-moderate physical activity that was not sufficient for them to lose weight, but drastically improved their insulin resistance and presumably long-term morbidity (Nassis et al. 2005; Denton et al. 2004). How does low-moderate physical activity exert such important effects on energy balance?

3 Energy Balance and Skeletal Muscle Metabolism

Skeletal muscle gives postural support, enables locomotion and is an important site for turnover of the carbon skeletons of amino acids, fatty acids and carbohydrates. Skeletal muscle therefore represents a key organ for intermediary metabolism; indeed, it accounts for about 40% of body mass, 20% of energy expenditure but 70–80% of insulin dependent glucose uptake (via glucose transporter 4 [GLUT4]) (Olefsky 1999). Skeletal muscle is comprised, basically, of primary and secondary fibres which, more importantly, may be subdivided into oxidative (i.e. support resting substrate level oxidation of primarily fatty acids and some glycogen) or glycolytic (i.e. primarily utilise locally stored glycogen for substrate-level oxidation).

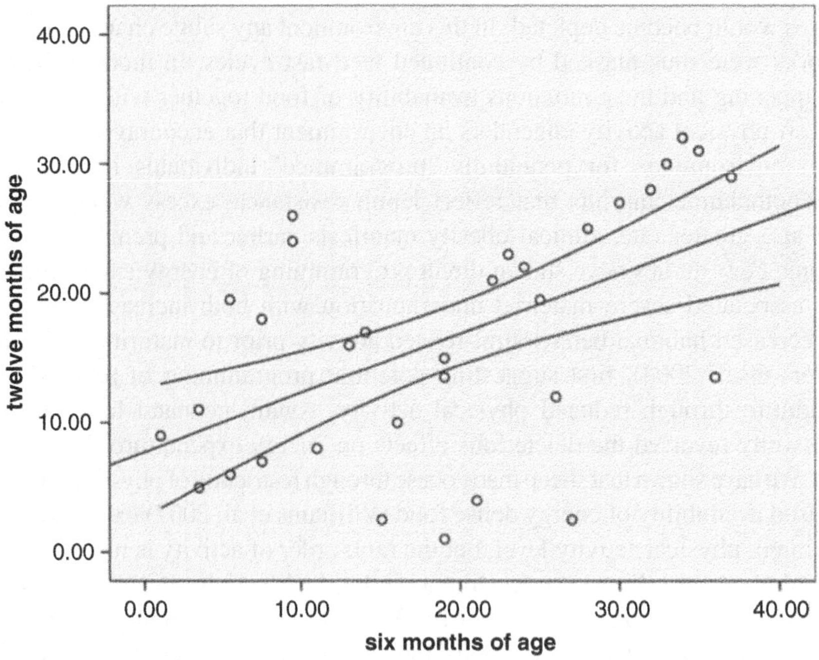

Fig. 1 Data for 24 h physical activity (accelerometry units) in all offspring were ranked after recording at 6 and 12 months of age. The slope of the correlation (with 95% CI) was statistically significant (r = 0.52; P = 0.002)

Primary fibre number appears unresponsive to environmental insults such as a poor prenatal diet i.e. they are largely genetically determined (Maltin et al. 2001; Fahey et al. 2005), but secondary fibres do appear susceptible (Daniel et al. 2007; Zhu et al. 2006; Mallinson et al. 2007). More importantly perhaps is that a prenatal limitation on the amount and activity of oxidative fibres has the potential to impact quite substantially on intermediary metabolism in adult life. For example, oxidative fibres express greater GLUT4 relative to glycolytic fibres (Duehlmeier et al. 2007; Daugaard et al. 2000), contain more mitochondria and subsequently more β oxidative enzymes such as carnitine parmitoyltransferase (CPT-1) (Zhu et al. 2006) and acetyl-CoA carboxylase, (ACC). Although muscle fibre number and type are fixed at birth (Maltin et al. 2001) subtle shifts in muscle oxidative capacity can be induced through activation of peroxisome proliferator activated receptor (PPAR) gamma coactivator alpha (PGC-1α) and beta (PGC-1β) (Arany et al. 2007) and adenosine monophosphate (AMP) activated protein kinase (AMPK) (Hardie et al. 2006) in response to physical activity.

Prenatal programming of skeletal muscle metabolism, physical activity and potentially even "intramuscular energy sensing" could have a significant influence on the predisposition to the facets of the metabolic syndrome induced by the *in utero* nutritional milieu. For example, a reduced overall capacity for fatty acid oxidation may pre-empt intramyocellular (ectopic) fatty acid deposition which has been implicated in the pathophysiology of Type 2 Diabetes (T2D; Roden 2005). Furthermore, (Wisloff et al. 2005) demonstrated a clear correlation between prenatally determined skeletal muscle oxidative capacity and cardiovascular health. Prenatal nutrient restriction has been shown to increase intracellular fatty acid deposition in the adult offspring of sheep (Zhu et al. 2006) and alter intracellular insulin signalling (Ozanne et al. 2005). Of course, with sufficient exercise-induced muscle contraction however, then such metabolic dysregulation is avoided by the activation of PGC-1α, PGC-1β (Hood et al. 2006; Mortensen et al. 2006) and AMPK (Hardie et al. 2006), leading to improvements in blood glucose clearance, glycogen production and fatty acid oxidation via mitochondrial biogenesis and increased expression of β-oxidative enzymes. Indeed over-expression of skeletal muscle specific PGC-1 confers resistance to T2D (Arany et al. 2007). As Chakravarthy and Booth hypothesised, low-moderate physical activity (or alternatively, the physiological recruitment of oxidative skeletal muscle fibres) appears to act as the gating mechanism for control of resting metabolism (Chakravarthy and Booth 2004).

4 Conclusion

Any early developmentally-induced compromise in the control of resting metabolism, either through deficits in oxidative fibre number or intramuscular energy sensing and handling could provide the initial trigger for increased susceptibility to the range of adverse symptoms that we associate with the metabolic syndrome; all that appears required to prevent these pathophysiological sequalae is regular low-moderate intensity exercise, irrespective of any reduction in bodyweight (Nassis et al. 2005; Denton et al. 2004). Perhaps the one easy, effective and economic health promotion initiative or intervention to be considered is prescription of exercise programs to overweight individuals and for those that have been *a priori* identified at particular risk i.e. the 'developmentally programmed', low birth weight-early growth acceleration infants.

Acknowledgements David S Gardner is funded through a British Heart Foundation Basic Science Lectureship and Philip Rhodes by a joint Medical Research Council and Institute of Clinical Research, University of Nottingham PhD studentship. The support of the European Union Sixth Framework Programme for Research and Technical Development of the European Community – The Early Nutrition Programming Project (FOOD-CT-2005-007036) is also acknowledged.

References

Arany, Z., Lebrasseur, N., Morris, C., Smith, E., Yang, W., Ma, Y., Chin, S., & Spiegelman, B. M. (2007). The transcriptional coactivator PGC-1beta drives the formation of oxidative type IIX fibers in skeletal muscle. *Cell Metab* **5**, 35–46.

Balthasar, N., Dalgaard, L. T., Lee, C. E., Yu, J., Funahashi, H., Williams, T., Ferreira, M., Tang, V., McGovern, R. A., Kenny, C. D., Christiansen, L. M., Edelstein, E., Choi, B., Boss, O., Aschkenasi, C., Zhang, C. Y., Mountjoy, K., Kishi, T., Elmquist, J. K., & Lowell, B. B. (2005). Divergence of melanocortin pathways in the control of food intake and energy expenditure. *Cell* **123**, 493–505.

Bedard, D., Shatenstein, B., & Nadon, S. (2004). Underreporting of energy intake from a self-administered food-frequency questionnaire completed by adults in Montreal. *Public Health Nutr* **7**, 675–681.

Bouret, S. G. & Simerly, R. B. (2006). Developmental programming of hypothalamic feeding circuits. *Clin Genet* **70**, 295–301.

Bouret, S. G., Draper, S. J., & Simerly, R. B. (2004). Trophic action of leptin on hypothalamic neurons that regulate feeding. *Science* **304**, 108–110.

Chakravarthy, M. V. & Booth, F. W. (2004). Eating, exercise, and "thrifty" genotypes: connecting the dots toward an evolutionary understanding of modern chronic diseases. *J Appl Physiol* **96**, 3–10.

Cripps, R. L., Martin-Gronert, M. S., & Ozanne, S. E. (2005). Fetal and perinatal programming of appetite. *Clin Sci (Lond)* **109**, 1–11.

Daniel, Z. C., Brameld, J. M., Craigon, J., Scollan, N. D., & Buttery, P. J. (2007). Effect of maternal dietary restriction during pregnancy on lamb carcass characteristics and muscle fiber composition. *J Anim Sci* **85**, 1565–1576.

Daugaard, J. R., Nielsen, J. N., Kristiansen, S., Andersen, J. L., Hargreaves, M., & Richter, E. A. (2000). Fiber type-specific expression of GLUT4 in human skeletal muscle: influence of exercise training. *Diabetes* **49**, 1092–1095.

Denton, J. C., Schultz, R., Jamurtas, A. Z., & Angelopoulos, T. J. (2004). Improvements in glucose tolerance in obese males with abnormal glucose tolerance following 10 days of aerobic exercise. *Prev Med* **38**, 885–888.

Duehlmeier, R., Sammet, K., Widdel, A., von Engelhardt, W., Wernery, U., Kinne, J., & Sallmann, H. P. (2007). Distribution patterns of the glucose transporters GLUT4 and GLUT1 in skeletal muscles of rats (Rattus norvegicus), pigs (Sus scrofa), cows (Bos taurus), adult goats, goat kids (Capra hircus), and camels (Camelus dromedarius). *Comp Biochem Physiol A Mol Integr Physiol* **146**, 274–282.

Enriori, P. J., Evans, A. E., Sinnayah, P., Jobst, E. E., Tonelli-Lemos, L., Billes, S. K., Glavas, M. M., Grayson, B. E., Perello, M., Nillni, E. A., Grove, K. L., & Cowley, M. A. (2007). Diet-induced obesity causes severe but reversible leptin resistance in arcuate melanocortin neurons. *Cell Metab* **5**, 181–194.

Fahey, A. J., Brameld, J. M., Parr, T., & Buttery, P. J. (2005). The effect of maternal undernutrition before muscle differentiation on the muscle fiber development of the newborn lamb. *J Anim Sci* **83**, 2564–2571.

Food Standards Agency & Department of Health (2004). National Diet and Nutrition Survey: adults aged 19–64 years. Krebs, J. and Johnson, M. **5**, 1–142. London, HMSO. Ref Type: Report.

Frayling, T. M., Timpson, N. J., Weedon, M. N., Zeggini, E., Freathy, R. M., Lindgren, C. M., Perry, J. R., Elliott, K. S., Lango, H., Rayner, N. W., Shields, B., Harries, L. W., Barrett, J. C., Ellard, S., Groves, C. J., Knight, B., Patch, A. M., Ness, A. R., Ebrahim, S., Lawlor, D. A., Ring, S. M., Ben Shlomo, Y., Jarvelin, M. R., Sovio, U., Bennett, A. J., Melzer, D., Ferrucci, L., Loos, R. J., Barroso, I., Wareham, N. J., Karpe, F., Owen, K. R., Cardon, L. R., Walker, M., Hitman, G. A., Palmer, C. N., Doney, A. S., Morris, A. D., Davey-Smith, G., Hattersley, A. T., & McCarthy, M. I. (2007). A common variant in the FTO gene is associated with body mass index and predisposes to childhood and adult obesity. *Science* **316**, 889–894.

Hardie, D. G., Hawley, S. A., & Scott, J. W. (2006). AMP-activated protein kinase – development of the energy sensor concept. *J Physiol* **574**, 7–15.

Hood, D. A., Irrcher, I., Ljubicic, V., & Joseph, A. M. (2006). Coordination of metabolic plasticity in skeletal muscle. *J Exp Biol* **209**, 2265–2275.

Horvath, T. L. & Bruning, J. C. (2006). Developmental programming of the hypothalamus: a matter of fat. *Nat Med* **12**, 52–53.

Kalra, S. P., Dube, M. G., Pu, S., Xu, B., Horvath, T. L., & Kalra, P. S. (1999). Interacting appetite-regulating pathways in the hypothalamic regulation of body weight. *Endocrinol Rev* **20**, 68–100.

Keith, S. W., Redden, D. T., Katzmarzyk, P. T., Boggiano, M. M., Hanlon, E. C., Benca, R. M., Ruden, D., Pietrobelli, A., Barger, J. L., Fontaine, K. R., Wang, C., Aronne, L. J., Wright, S. M., Baskin, M., Dhurandhar, N. V., Lijoi, M. C., Grilo, C. M., Deluca, M., Westfall, A. O., & Allison, D. B. (2006). Putative contributors to the secular increase in obesity: exploring the roads less traveled. *Int J Obes (Lond)* **30**, 1585–1594.

Kimm, S. Y., Glynn, N. W., Obarzanek, E., Kriska, A. M., Daniels, S. R., Barton, B. A., & Liu, K. (2005). Relation between the changes in physical activity and body-mass index during adolescence: a multicentre longitudinal study. *Lancet* **366**, 301–307.

Langley-Evans, S. C., Bellinger, L., & McMullen, S. (2005). Animal models of programming: early life influences on appetite and feeding behaviour. *Matern Child Nutr* **1**, 142–148.

Levine, J. A., Lanningham-Foster, L. M., McCrady, S. K., Krizan, A. C., Olson, L. R., Kane, P. H., Jensen, M. D., & Clark, M. M. (2005). Interindividual variation in posture allocation: possible role in human obesity. *Science* **307**, 584–586.

Lisboa, P. C., Passos, M. C., Dutra, S. C., Bonomo, I. T., Denolato, A. T., Reis, A. M., & Moura, E. G. (2006). Leptin and prolactin, but not corticosterone, modulate body weight and thyroid function in protein-malnourished lactating rats. *Horm Metab Res* **38**, 295–299.

Lissner, L. (2002). Measuring food intake in studies of obesity. *Public Health Nutr* **5**, 889–892.

Mallinson, J. E., Sculley, D. V., Craigon, J., Plant, R., Langley-Evans, S. C., & Brameld, J. M. (2007). Fetal exposure to a maternal low-protein diet during mid-gestation results in muscle-specific effects on fibre type composition in young rats. *Brit J Nutr* **98**, 292–299.

Maltin, C. A., Delday, M. I., Sinclair, K. D., Steven, J., & Sneddon, A. A. (2001). Impact of manipulations of myogenesis in utero on the performance of adult skeletal muscle. *Reproduction* **122**, 359–374.

Mark, A. L., Rahmouni, K., Correia, M., & Haynes, W. G. (2003). A leptin-sympathetic-leptin feedback loop: potential implications for regulation of arterial pressure and body fat. *Acta Physiol Scand* **177**, 345–349.

Miralles, O., Sanchez, J., Palou, A., & Pico, C. (2006). A physiological role of breast milk leptin in body weight control in developing infants. *Obesity (Silver.Spring)* **14**, 1371–1377.

Mortensen, O. H., Frandsen, L., Schjerling, P., Nishimura, E., & Grunnet, N. (2006). PGC-1alpha and PGC-1beta have both similar and distinct effects on myofiber switching toward an oxidative phenotype. *Am J Physiol Endocrinol Metab* **291**, E807–E816.

Mostyn, A., Sebert, S., Litten, J. C., Perkins, K. S., Laws, J., Symonds, M. E., & Clarke, L. (2006). Influence of porcine genotype on the abundance of thyroid hormones and leptin in sow milk and its impact on growth, metabolism and expression of key adipose tissue genes in offspring. *J Endocrinol* **190**, 631–639.

Muhlhausler, B. S., Adam, C. L., Findlay, P. A., Duffield, J. A., & McMillen, I. C. (2006). Increased maternal nutrition alters development of the appetite-regulating network in the brain. *FASEB J* **20**, 1257–1259.

Nassis, G. P., Papantakou, K., Skenderi, K., Triandafillopoulou, M., Kavouras, S. A., Yannakoulia, M., Chrousos, G. P., & Sidossis, L. S. (2005). Aerobic exercise training improves insulin sensitivity without changes in body weight, body fat, adiponectin, and inflammatory markers in overweight and obese girls. *Metabolism* **54**, 1472–1479.

National Food Survey (2007). Household food expenditure and consumption and nutrient intake 1974–2007. DEFRA/ONS (2007) Expenditure and Food Survey. TSO, London. https://statistics.defra.gov.uk/esg/publications/efs

Olefsky, J. M. (1999). Insulin-stimulated glucose transport minireview series. *J Biol Chem* **274**, 1863.

Oscai, L. B. & McGarr, J. A. (1978). Evidence that the amount of food consumed in early life fixes appetite in the rat. *Am J Physiol* **235**, R141–R144.

Ozanne, S. E., Jensen, C. B., Tingey, K. J., Storgaard, H., Madsbad, S., & Vaag, A. A. (2005). Low birth weight is associated with specific changes in muscle insulin signaling protein expression. *Diabetologia* **48**, 547–552.

Popkin, B. M. (2006). Global nutrition dynamics: the world is shifting rapidly toward a diet linked with noncommunicable diseases. *Am J Clin Nutr* **84**, 289–298.

Prentice, A. M. & Jebb, S. A. (2003). Fast foods, energy density and obesity: a possible mechanistic link. *Obes Rev* **4**, 187–194.

Prynne, C. J., Paul, A. A., Price, G. M., Day, K. C., Hilder, W. S., & Wadsworth, M. E. (1999). Food and nutrient intake of a national sample of 4-year-old children in 1950: comparison with the 1990s. *Public Health Nutr* **2**, 537–547.

Roden, M. (2005). Muscle triglycerides and mitochondrial function: possible mechanisms for the development of type 2 diabetes. *Int J Obes (Lond)* **29**(Suppl 2), S111–S115.

Savino, F., Liguori, S. A., Oggero, R., Silvestro, L., & Miniero, R. (2006). Maternal BMI and serum leptin concentration of infants in the first year of life. *Acta Paediatr* **95**, 414–418.

Smyth, S. & Heron, A. (2006). Diabetes and obesity: the twin epidemics. *Nat Med* **12**, 75–80.

Sothern, M. S. (2004). Obesity prevention in children: physical activity and nutrition. *Nutrition* **20**, 704–708.

Swinburn, B. & Egger, G. (2004). The runaway weight gain train: too many accelerators, not enough brakes. *BMJ* **329**, 736–739.

Vickers, M. H., Breier, B. H., Cutfield, W. S., Hofman, P. L., & Gluckman, P. D. (2000). Fetal origins of hyperphagia, obesity, and hypertension and postnatal amplification by hypercaloric nutrition. *Am J Physiol Endocrinol Metab* **279**, E83–E87.

Vickers, M. H., Breier, B. H., McCarthy, D., & Gluckman, P. D. (2003). Sedentary behavior during postnatal life is determined by the prenatal environment and exacerbated by postnatal hypercaloric nutrition. *Am J Physiol Regul Integr Comp Physiol* **285**, R271–R273.

Vickers, M. H., Gluckman, P. D., Coveny, A. H., Hofman, P. L., Cutfield, W. S., Gertler, A., Breier, B. H., & Harris, M. (2005). Neonatal leptin treatment reverses developmental programming. *Endocrinology* **146**, 4211–4216.

Widdowson, E. M. (1970). Harmony of growth. *Lancet* **1**, 902–905.

Widdowson, E. M. & McCance, R. A. (1975). A review: new thoughts on growth. *Pediatr Res* **9**, 154–156.

Wilkin, T. J., Mallam, K. M., Metcalf, B. S., Jeffery, A. N., & Voss, L. D. (2006). Variation in physical activity lies with the child, not his environment: evidence for an 'activitystat' in young children (EarlyBird 16). *Int J Obes (Lond)* **30**, 1050–1055.

Williams, P. J., Kurlak, L. O., Perkins, A. C., Budge, H., Stephenson, T., Keisler, D., Symonds, M. E., & Gardner, D. S. (2007). Hypertension and impaired renal function accompany juvenile obesity: the effect of prenatal diet. *Kidney Int* **72**(3), 279–289.
Wisloff, U., Najjar, S. M., Ellingsen, O., Haram, P. M., Swoap, S., Al Share, Q., Fernstrom, M., Rezaei, K., Lee, S. J., Koch, L. G., & Britton, S. L. (2005). Cardiovascular risk factors emerge after artificial selection for low aerobic capacity. *Science* **307**, 418–420.
Zhu, M. J., Ford, S. P., Means, W. J., Hess, B. W., Nathanielsz, P. W., & Du, M. (2006). Maternal nutrient restriction affects properties of skeletal muscle in offspring. *J Physiol* **575**, 241–250.

Nutrient–Gene Interactions in Early Life Programming: Leptin in Breast Milk Prevents Obesity Later on in Life

Andreu Palou, Juana Sánchez, and Catalina Picó

Abstract Breast milk is practically the only food eaten during the first months of life in fully breastfed infants and it is assumed to match the nutritional needs during these first months of postnatal life. Breastfeeding compared with infant formula feeding confers protection against several metabolic and physiological changes later on in life and, particularly, against obesity and related medical complications. Recent data from our laboratory, identifying leptin as the first specific compound responsible for these beneficial effects, are reviewed and discussed.

Keywords Breastfeeding • obesity • leptin

Abbreviations BMI: body mass index; CCK: cholecystokinin; HF: high-fat diet; NF: normal fat diet; OB-Rb: leptin receptor; NPY: neuropeptide Y; POMC: pro-opiomelanocortin; SOCS-3: suppressor of cytokine signaling 3

1 Introduction

The basis of our health, well-being and longevity is much related to the biochemical diversity of the foods we eat. In particular, early life feeding may strongly influence later health outcomes (Barker et al. 2002; Novak 2002). Epidemiological studies over the past 20 years have shown how changes in maternal food intake during fetal growth and feeding during early postnatal development affect susceptibility to cardiovascular disease, obesity, type II diabetes, osteoporosis and other problems and patterns in adult life (e.g. Ong and Dunger 2004; Remacle et al. 2004; Novak et al. 2006;

A. Palou(✉), J. Sánchez, and C. Picó
Laboratory of Molecular Biology, Nutrition and Biotechnology (Nutrigenomics), University of the Balearic Islands (UIB) and CIBER Fisiopatología de la Obesidad y Nutrición (CIBEROBN), Palma de Mallorca 07122, Spain
andreu.palou@uib.es

B. Koletzko et al. (eds.), *Early Nutrition Programming and Health Outcomes in Later Life: Obesity and Beyond*,

Valsamakis et al. 2006). As deduced from animal or *in vitro* studies, differences are caused by the interaction of food components or other environmental factors with our chromosomes allowing the imprinting of metabolic schemes in individuals (epigenetics) that may confer a different susceptibility to alterations later on in life (Levin 2000).

Breast milk is practically the only food eaten during the first months of life in fully breastfed infants and, compared with artificial infant formula milk, it confers protection against several metabolic and physiological changes later on in life (von Kries et al. 1999; Gillman et al. 2001; Armstrong and Reilly 2002; Harder et al. 2005). Human milk provided by healthy mothers is believed to cover the infant's nutrient requirements during the first half year of life or more. It is a mixture of biomolecules, some of them having been traditionally recognized as nutrients, together with others – such as leptin – for which a function has still to be determined. Bioactive components in milk may have relevant physiological effects in the neonate infant that could be apparent both in the short- and medium-term as well as later on in life and in ageing. Human milk composition has a dynamic nature and varies with time during postpartum: it can be affected by the mother's diet, various diseases and other environmental factors, while the changes of milk composition with duration of lactation is assumed to match the changing needs of the growing infant over time (Kunz et al. 1999). In particular, milk is a source of individual peptides and proteins that potentially may benefit the breastfeeding infant either in the short-term or later on. Nowadays a key challenge in research is to progressively unveil the nexus between milk components and health/disease outcomes later in life, including the identification of the involved bioactive components and their mechanisms of action. Early identification may be the way to prevent, for example, the formation of permanent neural connections that promote and perpetuate obesity in individuals (Levin 2000). Questions such as the optimal range of levels of these compounds in artificial infant formula, or how they could be optimized in breast milk by encouraging appropriate diets and/or life style conditions for mothers, appear as paramount importance.

Studies developed in recent years in our laboratory have allowed us to discover a novel function for one of these proteins that is naturally present in human breast milk and not in infant formula. This protein is leptin, a new function of which during lactation is to confer protection against the later development of overweight and other associated medical complications.

2 Previously Known Functions of Leptin

The cloning of the gene that codifies for leptin (Zhang et al. 1994) opened a new window to understanding the system that controls body weight in mammals. Leptin is a hormone primarily produced and secreted by the adipose tissue, and its circulating levels correlate with the size of fat stores (Maffei et al. 1995; Ostlund et al. 1996). Leptin signals nutritional status and energy storage levels to feeding centers in the hypothalamus and other central areas, through its action on the expression and release of orexigenic and anorexigenic neuropeptides, including, respectively, neuropeptide Y (NPY) and pro-opiomelanocortin (POMC). In the arcuate nucleus, NPY and POMC neurons express the long form of leptin receptor (OB-Rb), which is functionally coupled to the Janus kinase-signal transducer and activator of transcription intracellular signaling cascade and produces an endogenous inhibitor (suppressor of cytokine signaling 3, SOCS-3) upon activation. This action prompts appropriate regulation of food intake and energy expenditure processes and, provided the system works well, helps our body to maintain the amount of fat stores within a certain range (Zhang et al. 1994; Ahima and Flier 2000). However, the vast majority of obese people appear to be resistant to the action of leptin. In fact, the administration of this hormone, while proven to be effective in reducing fat and normalizing metabolic disorders in leptin-deficient mice and humans, has not proven to be effective in most cases of obesity (Halaas et al. 1995; Pelleymounter et al. 1995; Farooqi et al. 1999).

3 Food Related Metabolic Programming

It is clear that mammalian development occurs in more or less defined stages. Human epidemiology suggests that specific nutrients, food intake patterns, and in general physiologic and metabolic alterations during prenatal and early postnatal development can affect susceptibility to various adult-onset chronic diseases, including obesity, cardiovascular disease, type-II diabetes, and hypertension (see Ong and Dunger 2004; Remacle et al. 2004; Novak et al. 2006; Valsamakis et al. 2006). Thus, the term metabolic imprinting describes the processes whereby cells have a biological memory for external influences that can be passed on to daughter cells (Waterland and Garza 1999). It involves the concept (Lucas 2000) that a stimulus or insult operating at a critical or sensitive period of development (the specific window of sensitivity) could result in a long-standing or life-long effect on the structure or function of the organism.

Metabolic imprinting on neural circuits and related processes involved in energy homeostasis during the perinatal period that can alter neuronal development may play an important role in setting the future patterns of body weight and fat gain in susceptible individuals (Levin 2000; Park 2005). Epigenetics refers to these stable alterations in gene expression that do not involve mutations of the DNA itself while conferring stable maintenance of a particular gene expression pattern through mitotic cell division (Holliday and Pugh 1975). Because the pattern of DNA methylation is both stable and heritable, it has been considered that methylation is the main epigenetic basis for imprinting, and good evidence supports this connection (see Jirtle and Weidman 2007). Histone proteins also contribute and it has been suggested that DNA methylation is connected mechanically to histone modification (Jirtle and Weidman 2007).

According to Waterland and Garza (Waterland and Garza 1999), metabolic imprinting encompasses adaptive responses to specific nutritional conditions early in life that are characterized by (1) susceptibility limited to a critical ontogenic period early in development (the critical window), (2) a persistent effect lasting into adulthood, (3) a specific and measurable outcome, and (4) a dose–response relationship between exposure and outcome.

Therefore, as subtle environmental influences during specific ontogenic periods can cause stable alterations in mammalian epigenotype, early intervention in mothers and infants may be the way to prevent the formation of persistent neural connections that promote and perpetuate obesity in predisposed individuals. However, our knowledge of the biology underlying metabolic imprinting or programming is fairly limited.

4 The Role of Leptin in Breast Milk

Leptin is produced by mammary epithelium (Smith-Kirwin et al. 1998) and is naturally present in breast milk (Casabiell et al. 1997; Houseknecht et al. 1997). Leptin concentrations in human milk vary significantly between people, and there is a positive correlation between leptin concentration in milk and maternal plasma leptin levels and adiposity (Houseknecht et al. 1997; Uysal et al. 2002; Miralles et al. 2006). Thus, breastfed infants nursed by mothers with significant adiposity may be exposed to higher amounts of leptin than infants nursed by lean mothers, and much higher than those fed with infant formulas, which do not have leptin as an ingredient (O'Connor et al. 2003).

4.1 Benefits of Breastfeeding Compared with Infant Formula Feeding: Could Any Specific Component Be Responsible?

There is increasing epidemiological evidence suggesting that breastfeeding compared with infant formula confers protection against obesity later in life (von Kries et al. 1999; Gillman et al. 2001; Armstrong and Reilly 2002; Harder et al. 2005). In addition, a meta-analysis of the existing studies on duration of breastfeeding and risk of overweight (Harder et al. 2005) strongly supports a dose-dependent association between longer duration of breastfeeding and decrease in risk of overweight. However causality has never been related to any specific compound of breast milk.

Bearing in mind that leptin is naturally present in human breast milk (Casabiell et al. 1997; Houseknecht et al. 1997) but is not present in infant formula (O'Connor et al. 2003), and our previous findings that, in neonate rats, orally taken leptin can be absorbed by the immature stomach and inhibits food intake (Oliver et al. 2002;

Sanchez et al. 2005), we suggested the hypothesis that programming by an early leptin-deficient diet may be a mechanism that links early nutrition with later obesity.

4.2 A Possible Physiological Role of Oral Leptin During Lactation

Although leptin is mainly produced by the adipose tissue, this hormone is also produced by other tissues, such as stomach (Bado et al. 1998; Cinti et al. 2000, 2001), placenta (Masuzaki et al. 1997), skeletal muscle (Wang et al. 1998), and mammary epithelium (Smith-Kirwin et al. 1998) and it is naturally present in maternal milk (Casabiell et al. 1997; Houseknecht et al. 1997). While leptin produced by the adipose tissue is known to play a main role in the chronic control of energy balance, the role of leptin produced by the stomach is less known and has been related to the short-term control of food intake, acting as a satiety signal (Cinti et al. 2001; Pico et al. 2003). There is evidence indicating that feeding stimulates the secretion of leptin by the stomach in humans (Cinti et al. 2000, 2001) and in rats (Bado et al. 1998; Pico et al. 2002), and pepsinogen secretagogues such as cholecystokinin (CCK), gastrin or secretin also induce gastric leptin release in rats (Bado et al. 1998). Leptin receptors are present in the human stomach (Breidert et al. 1999) and in the mouse gastrointestinal tract (Morton et al. 1998), and additionally leptin is capable of direct acute activation of vagal afferent neurons that originate in the gastric and intestinal walls and terminate in the nucleus tractus solitarius (Yuan et al. 1999), providing rapid information to the brain.

Interestingly, in human subjects, it has been shown that leptin is released in response to food intake (Cinti et al. 2000): one of the patients in this study, who did not follow the required fasting for endoscopy, had much lower immunostaining for leptin in the gastric cells compared with individuals who had fasted overnight. In rats, gastric leptin is also mobilized in response to food intake (Bado et al. 1998; Pico et al. 2002). A short food intake stimulus (20 min of refeeding) following fasting is capable of practically emptying the leptin stores from within the stomach mucosa (Pico et al. 2002).

Given the unknown properties of gastric leptin, the fact that this hormone is sensitive to the nutritional state, being rapidly mobilized in response to food intake following fasting or after the administration of satiety factors, suggests a role for this protein in the short-term regulation of feeding. On the other hand, no previous insights on potential effects of leptin in the long-term were available.

However, it was reported that leptin supplied by milk, or leptin supplied as a water solution, can be absorbed by the immature stomach of suckling rats (Casabiell et al. 1997; Oliver et al. 2002; Sanchez et al. 2005) and be transferred to the bloodstream (Casabiell et al. 1997; Sanchez et al. 2005), suggesting that maternal milk leptin may play a regulatory role during development. We evaluated the effects of the administration of an acute oral dose of leptin on food intake in neonatal rats as well as the prolonged effects of the chronic administration of a daily oral dose of leptin, close to physiological levels, during the suckling period on the gastric leptin system and energy balance, to determine the importance of leptin supplied by maternal milk during lactation (Sanchez et al. 2005). Leptin supplied from maternal milk appeared to be the main source of leptin in the stomach during the suckling period, particularly during the first half of this period, in which gastric leptin production is kept low (Oliver et al. 2002). This exogenous leptin could exert biological effects in neonates at a time in which both the adipose tissue and appetite regulatory systems are immature (Yuan et al. 1999). Of interest, the administration of physiological oral doses of leptin during the suckling period was shown to inhibit food intake, but without affecting body weight gain during this period (Sanchez et al. 2005). It was concluded that leptin exerts important effects in a physiologically regulated manner during early postnatal life, in the neonatal control of energy balance and possibly in other functions during development (Sanchez et al. 2005).

4.3 Evidence for a Protective Effect of Oral Leptin During Lactation on Later Obesity

Because of (i) epidemiological evidence suggesting that breastfeeding compared with infant formula provides protection against obesity later in life (Armstrong and Reilly 2002), and (ii) bearing in mind that leptin is naturally present in the human breast milk (Casabiell et al. 1997) but not present in infant formula (O'Connor et al. 2003), and (iii) our previous findings showing that orally taken leptin by neonate rats can be absorbed by the immature stomach and inhibits food intake (Sanchez et al. 2005), we suggested the hypothesis that leptin could be the specific compound (or at least one of them) responsible of the beneficial effects of breast milk in providing protection against later obesity.

To test this hypothesis, we performed a study in rats to evaluate whether supplementation with physiological doses of oral leptin during lactation could have long-term effects on body weight regulation (Pico et al. 2007). Thus, a daily oral dose of leptin (equivalent to five times the amount of leptin ingested normally from maternal milk during the suckling period) or just the vehicle was given to suckling male rats during lactation, and animals were fed after weaning with a normal fat (NF) or a high-fat (HF) diet until the age of 6 months. Results showed that leptin-treated animals had, in adulthood, lower body weight and fat content and ate fewer calories than their untreated controls, under both NF and HF diets. Unlike adipocitary leptin production, adult animals that were leptin-treated during lactation displayed higher gastric leptin production and secretion, without changes in OB-Rb mRNA levels, suggesting that short-term control of food intake mediated by gastric leptin was more active in leptin-treated animals, and this could be partially responsible for their lower food intake. At the hypothalamic level, differences in neuropeptide expression – particularly in the main neuropeptides involved in the anorexigenic action of leptin, NPY, with orexigenic activity, and POMC, with anorexigenic activity – could also contribute to explain the lower food intake in leptin-treated rats, compared with their untreated controls. In particular, in response to HF diet, we found that leptin-treated animals (contrary to controls) showed lower hypothalamic NPY/POMC mRNA ratio. Of note, hypothalamic OB-Rb mRNA levels decreased in control animals as an effect of HF diet feeding but remained unchanged in leptin-treated animals, probably reflecting the higher resistance to obesity development of leptin-treated animals. In addition, SOCS-3 mRNA levels were lower in leptin-treated animals than in their controls, both under normal or HF diet. Bearing in mind that SOCS-3 is a leptin-inducible inhibitor of leptin signaling and a potential mediator of leptin resistance in obesity (Bjorbaek et al. 1998), the reduction of its expression in leptin-treated animals might be enough to both increase leptin action and to attenuate sensitivity to diet-induced obesity.

The overall conclusion was that animals that received leptin during lactation became more protected against fat accumulation in adult life and seemed to be more sensitive to the short- and long-term regulation of food intake by leptin (Pico et al. 2007). Thus, leptin plays an important role in the earlier stages of neonatal life, as a component of breast milk, in the prevention of later obesity. Others studies have confirmed these results under different food and long term conditions.

4.4 Evidence in Humans

To obtain some evidence in humans, a group of 28 non-obese women (BMI between 16.3 and 27.3 kg/m^2) who breastfed their infants for at least 6 months and their infants were studied (Miralles et al. 2006). We found that, during the whole lactation period, milk leptin concentration correlated positively with maternal plasma leptin concentration and with maternal BMI. In addition, milk leptin concentration at 1 month of lactation was negatively correlated with infant BMI at 18 and 24 months of age. A better negative correlation was also found between log milk leptin concentration at 1 and at 3 months of lactation and infant BMI from 12 to 24 months of age. We concluded that, at least in non-obese mothers, infant body weight during the first 2 years may be influenced by milk leptin concentration during the first stages of lactation. Thus, moderate milk-borne maternal leptin appears to provide moderate protection to infants from an excess of weight gain (Miralles et al. 2006).

5 Conclusions

All in all, the results obtained in non-obese mothers and their infants (Miralles et al. 2006) together with those showing the mechanistic evidence obtained in rats (Pico et al. 2007) suggest that milk leptin is an important factor that could explain, at least partially, the increased risk of obesity of formula-fed infants with respect to breastfed infants as found in epidemiologic studies. It also opens a new area of research on both the use of leptin in the design of more appropriate infant formula as well as the research on different factors that control leptin levels in maternal milk.

Acknowledgements Spanish Government (grants AGL 2004-07496/ALI and AGL2006-04887/ALI). Our Laboratory is a member of the European Research Network of Excellence NuGO (The European Nutrigenomics Organization, EU Contract: n° FP6-506360).

References

Ahima, R. S. and J. S. Flier (2000). "Leptin." *Annu Rev Physiol* **62**: 413–437.

Armstrong, J. and J. J. Reilly (2002). "Breastfeeding and lowering the risk of childhood obesity." *Lancet* **359**(9322): 2003–2004.

Bado, A., S. Levasseur, S. Attoub, S. Kermorgant, J. P. Laigneau, M. N. Bortoluzzi, L. Moizo, T. Lehy, M. Guerre-Millo, Y. Le Marchand-Brustel and M. J. Lewin (1998). "The stomach is a source of leptin." *Nature* **394**(6695): 790–793.

Barker, D. J., J. G. Eriksson, T. Forsen and C. Osmond (2002). "Fetal origins of adult disease: strength of effects and biological basis." *Int J Epidemiol* **31**(6): 1235–1239.

Bjorbaek, C., J. K. Elmquist, J. D. Frantz, S. E. Shoelson and J. S. Flier (1998). "Identification of SOCS-3 as a potential mediator of central leptin resistance." *Mol Cell* **1**(4): 619–625.

Breidert, M., S. Miehlke, A. Glasow, Z. Orban, M. Stolte, G. Ehninger, E. Bayerdorffer, O. Nettesheim, U. Halm, A. Haidan and S. R. Bornstein (1999). "Leptin and its receptor in normal human gastric mucosa and in Helicobacter pylori-associated gastritis." *Scand J Gastroenterol* **34**(10): 954–961.

Casabiell, X., V. Pineiro, M. A. Tome, R. Peino, C. Dieguez and F. F. Casanueva (1997). "Presence of leptin in colostrum and/or breast milk from lactating mothers: a potential role in the regulation of neonatal food intake." *J Clin Endocrinol Metab* **82**(12): 4270–4273.

Cinti, S., R. D. Matteis, C. Pico, E. Ceresi, A. Obrador, C. Maffeis, J. Oliver and A. Palou (2000). "Secretory granules of endocrine and chief cells of human stomach mucosa contain leptin." *Int J Obes Relat Metab Disord* **24**(6): 789–793.

Cinti, S., R. de Matteis, E. Ceresi, C. Pico, J. Oliver, P. Oliver, A. Palou, A. Obrador and C. Maffeis (2001). "Leptin in the human stomach." *Gut* **49**(1): 155.

Farooqi, I. S., S. A. Jebb, G. Langmack, E. Lawrence, C. H. Cheetham, A. M. Prentice, I. A. Hughes, M. A. McCamish and S. O'Rahilly (1999). "Effects of recombinant leptin therapy in a child with congenital leptin deficiency." *N Engl J Med* **341**(12): 879–884.

Gillman, M. W., S. L. Rifas-Shiman, C. A. Camargo, Jr., C. S. Berkey, A. L. Frazier, H. R. Rockett, A. E. Field and G. A. Colditz (2001). "Risk of overweight among adolescents who were breastfed as infants." *JAMA* **285**(19): 2461–2467.

Halaas, J. L., K. S. Gajiwala, M. Maffei, S. L. Cohen, B. T. Chait, D. Rabinowitz, R. L. Lallone, S. K. Burley and J. M. Friedman (1995). "Weight-reducing effects of the plasma protein encoded by the obese gene." *Science* **269**(5223): 543–546.

Harder, T., R. Bergmann, G. Kallischnigg and A. Plagemann (2005). "Duration of breastfeeding and risk of overweight: a meta-analysis." *Am J Epidemiol* **162**(5): 397–403.

Holliday, R. and J. E. Pugh (1975). "DNA modification mechanisms and gene activity during development." *Science* **187**(4173): 226–232.

Houseknecht, K. L., M. K. McGuire, C. P. Portocarrero, M. A. McGuire and K. Beerman (1997). "Leptin is present in human milk and is related to maternal plasma leptin concentration and adiposity." *Biochem Biophys Res Commun* **240**(3): 742–747.

Jirtle, R. L. and J. R. Weidman (2007). "Imprinted and more equal." *Am Sci* **95**: 143–149.

Kunz, C., M. Rodriguez-Palmero, B. Koletzko and R. Jensen (1999). "Nutritional and biochemical properties of human milk, Part I: general aspects, proteins, and carbohydrates." *Clin Perinatol* **26**(2): 307–333.

Levin, B. E. (2000). "The obesity epidemic: metabolic imprinting on genetically susceptible neural circuits." *Obes Res* **8**(4): 342–347.

Lucas, A. (2000). "Programming not metabolic imprinting." *Am J Clin Nutr* **71**(2): 602.

Maffei, M., J. Halaas, E. Ravussin, R. E. Pratley, G. H. Lee, Y. Zhang, H. Fei, S. Kim, R. Lallone, S. Ranganathan, P. A. Kern and J. M. Friedman (1995). "Leptin levels in human and rodent: measurement of plasma leptin and ob RNA in obese and weight-reduced subjects." *Nat Med* **1**(11): 1155–1161.

Masuzaki, H., Y. Ogawa, N. Sagawa, K. Hosoda, T. Matsumoto, H. Mise, H. Nishimura, Y. Yoshimasa, I. Tanaka, T. Mori and K. Nakao (1997). "Nonadipose tissue production of leptin: leptin as a novel placenta-derived hormone in humans." *Nat Med* **3**(9): 1029–1033.

Miralles, O., J. Sanchez, A. Palou and C. Pico (2006). "A physiological role of breast milk leptin in body weight control in developing infants." *Obesity (Silver Spring)* **14**(8): 1371–1377.

Morton, N. M., V. Emilsson, Y. L. Liu and M. A. Cawthorne (1998). "Leptin action in intestinal cells." *J Biol Chem* **273**(40): 26194–26201.

Novak, D. (2002). "Nutrition in early life. How important is it?" *Clin Perinatol* **29**(2): 203–223.

Novak, D. A., M. Desai and M. G. Ross (2006). "Gestational programming of offspring obesity/hypertension." *J Matern Fetal Neonatal Med* **19**(10): 591–599.

O'Connor, D., V. Funanage, R. Locke, M. Spear and K. Leef (2003). "Leptin is not present in infant formulas." *J Endocrinol Invest* **26**(5): 490.

Oliver, P., C. Pico, R. De Matteis, S. Cinti and A. Palou (2002). "Perinatal expression of leptin in rat stomach." *Dev Dyn* **223**(1): 148–154.

Ong, K. K. and D. B. Dunger (2004). "Birth weight, infant growth and insulin resistance." *Eur J Endocrinol* **151**(Suppl 3): U131–U139.

Ostlund, R. E., Jr., J. W. Yang, S. Klein and R. Gingerich (1996). "Relation between plasma leptin concentration and body fat, gender, diet, age, and metabolic covariates." *J Clin Endocrinol Metab* **81**(11): 3909–3913.

Park, C. S. (2005). "Role of compensatory mammary growth in epigenetic control of gene expression." *FASEB J* **19**(12): 1586–1591.

Pelleymounter, M. A., M. J. Cullen, M. B. Baker, R. Hecht, D. Winters, T. Boone and F. Collins (1995). "Effects of the obese gene product on body weight regulation in ob/ob mice." *Science* **269**(5223): 540–543.

Pico, C., J. Sanchez, P. Oliver and A. Palou (2002). "Leptin production by the stomach is upregulated in obese (fa/fa) Zucker rats." *Obes Res* **10**(9): 932–938.

Pico, C., P. Oliver, J. Sanchez and A. Palou (2003). "Gastric leptin: a putative role in the short-term regulation of food intake." *Brit J Nutr* **90**(4): 735–741.

Pico, C., P. Oliver, J. Sanchez, O. Miralles, A. Caimari, T. Priego and A. Palou (2007). "The intake of physiological doses of leptin during lactation in rats prevents obesity in later life." *Int J Obes (Lond)* **31**(8): 1199–1209.

Remacle, C., F. Bieswal and B. Reusens (2004). "Programming of obesity and cardiovascular disease." *Int J Obes Relat Metab Disord* **28**(Suppl 3): S46–S53.

Sanchez, J., P. Oliver, O. Miralles, E. Ceresi, C. Pico and A. Palou (2005). "Leptin orally supplied to neonate rats is directly uptaken by the immature stomach and may regulate short-term feeding." *Endocrinology* **146**(6): 2575–2582.

Smith-Kirwin, S. M., D. M. O'Connor, J. De Johnston, E. D. Lancey, S. G. Hassink and V. L. Funanage (1998). "Leptin expression in human mammary epithelial cells and breast milk." *J Clin Endocrinol Metab* **83**(5): 1810–1813.

Uysal, F. K., E. E. Onal, Y. Z. Aral, B. Adam, U. Dilmen and Y. Ardicolu (2002). "Breast milk leptin: its relationship to maternal and infant adiposity." *Clin Nutr* **21**(2): 157–160.

Valsamakis, G., C. Kanaka-Gantenbein, A. Malamitsi-Puchner and G. Mastorakos (2006). "Causes of intrauterine growth restriction and the postnatal development of the metabolic syndrome." *Ann N Y Acad Sci* **1092**: 138–147.

von Kries, R., B. Koletzko, T. Sauerwald, E. von Mutius, D. Barnert, V. Grunert and H. von Voss (1999). "Breast feeding and obesity: cross sectional study." *BMJ* **319**(7203): 147–150.

Wang, J., R. Liu, M. Hawkins, N. Barzilai and L. Rossetti (1998). “A nutrient-sensing pathway regulates leptin gene expression in muscle and fat.” *Nature* **393**(6686): 684–688.
Waterland, R. A. and C. Garza (1999). “Potential mechanisms of metabolic imprinting that lead to chronic disease.” *Am J Clin Nutr* **69**(2): 179–197.
Yuan, C. S., A. S. Attele, J. A. Wu, L. Zhang and Z. Q. Shi (1999). “Peripheral gastric leptin modulates brain stem neuronal activity in neonates.” *Am J Physiol* **277**(3 Pt 1): G626–G630.
Zhang, Y., R. Proenca, M. Maffei, M. Barone, L. Leopold and J. M. Friedman (1994). “Positional cloning of the mouse obese gene and its human homologue.” *Nature* **372**(6505): 425–432.

Early Nutrition and Later Obesity: Animal Models Provide Insights into Mechanisms

Cornelia C. Metges

Abstract Epidemiological evidence suggests that *in utero* as well as early postnatal life exposure to an imbalanced nutrition are both related to a greater propensity to become obese in later life. Rodent and sheep models of metabolic programming of obesity by early life nutrition include maternal low and high dietary protein and energy or food intake as well as high fat diets. Maternal nutritional imbalance during pregnancy and/or lactation programs energy expenditure, food intake and physical activity in the offspring. Underlying mechanisms of altered energy balance in programmed offspring are associated with disturbances of ontogeny of hypothalamic feeding circuits, leptin and glucocorticoid action which have long-lasting effects on food intake, energy expenditure and fat tissue metabolism.

Keywords Metabolic programming • obesity • animal model • leptin • glucocorticoids

Abbreviations ARH: hypothalamic arcuate nucleus; 11ßHSD1: 11ß-hydroxysteroid dehydrogenase type 1; MLP: maternal low protein; mRNA: messenger RNA; GR: glucocorticoid receptor; UN: undernutrition

1 Introduction

It is now increasingly recognized that *in utero* as well as early postnatal life exposure to an imbalanced nutrition are both related to a greater propensity to become obese in later life. Babies small at birth showing high catch-up growth rates have a higher risk of becoming obese in later life (Okosun et al. 2000; Ong 2006). Catch-up growth in early infancy is associated with a high intake of energy

C.C. Metges
Research Institute of Farm Animal Biology, Research unit 'Nutritional Physiology', Wilhelm-Stahl-Allee 2, 18196 Dummerstorf, Germany
metges@fbn-dummerstorf.de; http://nutrition.fbn-dummerstorf.de

B. Koletzko et al. (eds.), *Early Nutrition Programming and Health Outcomes in Later Life: Obesity and Beyond*,

and macronutrients via formula feeding during the first weeks of life (Owen et al. 2005; Stettler et al. 2005; Kensara et al. 2007). In addition, babies born to obese mothers or mothers with gestational diabetes are more likely to be large for gestational age and become obese later in life (Dörner and Plagemann 1994; Levin and Govek 1998; Boney et al. 2005).

These observations are in keeping with the 'predictive adaptive response' hypothesis (Gluckman and Hanson 2004), an extension of the Hales 'thrifty phenotype' hypothesis (Hales and Barker 1992). According to this, an inadequate *in utero* nutritional environment is signalled to the fetus by maternal/placental circulating hormones or metabolites to which the fetal organism adapts, thereby predicting the postnatal nutritional plane in order to maximise the chances of survival. If the nutritional environment after birth is similarly poor, the *in utero* adjustment confers an advantage. When exposed to affluent nutritional conditions the degree of mismatch between the pre- and postnatal environments is a determinant of subsequent disorder.

It is unclear to what extent the world's obesity epidemic can be explained by its developmental origin (Keith et al. 2006). Due to its public health relevance it is important, however, to understand the mechanisms underlying the early life origin of obesity.

2 Animal Models

Although animal studies have provided insights into mechanisms of the association between maternal nutritional imbalance during pregnancy and lactation and offspring obesity, there are limitations of these models for the situation in the human species. Due to their short lifespan and moderate housing requirements rodents have been frequently used to model some of the epidemiological observations and conditions in humans. However, although both human and rat offspring are born helpless, the largest limitation of the rodent model lies in the difference of timing in CNS development (Clancy et al. 2001). In regard to brain development the approximate equivalent of a human neonate is a rat pup at age 12–13 days (reviewed in Watson et al. 2006). In contrast to humans, the CNS is relatively mature at birth in the guinea pig and ungulates (Watson et al. 2006). Another recognized animal model is the sheep in which effects of maternal global under- and overnutrition on health consequences have been determined (Wallace et al. 2004; Symonds et al. 2004; Metges and Hammon 2005). The sheep, in contrast to rodents, resembles human pregnancies which are singleton or twin in that there are large similarities in the endocrine environment in the periparturient period and the ontogeny of fetal adipose deposition (Symonds et al. 2003, 2004). Due to their size, experimental handling and blood sampling are easier in sheep than in rodents but their longer lifespan protracts the exploration of long-term health consequences of early nutrition.

2.1 *Metabolic Programming of Obesity by Early Life Nutrition in Animal Models*

It is interesting to note that a frequently used rodent maternal low protein (MLP) model (50% of control dietary protein) known to cause fetal growth retardation (Langley-Evans 2000) does not always result in low birth weight offspring (Bellinger et al. 2006). Only very few studies report obesity and catch-up growth in the offspring which seems to, however, always require postnatal overnutrition (Ozanne and Hales 2004; Petry et al. 1997). Mice and rat offspring only exposed to a MLP diet *in utero* do not become obese (Bellinger et al. 2006). Reasons for different results among protein-restriction studies are likely related to differences in animal genotype, dietary composition, and the ontogenetic time window of nutritional insult (Langley-Evans 2000; Armitage et al. 2004; Cherala et al. 2006). In the sheep, consequences for adipose tissue deposition are dependent on the timing of maternal nutrient restriction during pregnancy (Symonds et al. 2004). Maternal undernutrition (UN) models characterized by reduction of ad libitum intake during pregnancy (30–70%), result in fetal growth retardation but not always in increased body weight or adiposity (Anguita et al. 1993; Vickers et al. 2000; Ozaki et al. 2001). Hypercaloric nutrition of offspring born to undernourished mothers post-weaning amplifies or is necessary for the development of adiposity (Vickers et al. 2000, 2003).

Intuitively one associates poor nutrition with a diet restricted in a specific component, such as protein, or energy. However, poor nutrition today can also be high-sugar and -fat diets or general overeating. In addition, due to the high contribution of meat and dairy products, protein intakes above requirements are also widespread and high protein diets are increasingly used to combat obesity or maintain reduced body weight (Westerterp-Plantenga 2003). Recently, maternal dietary protein intake was reported to be inversely related to birth weight and ponderal index (Andreasyan et al. 2007). We and others have shown earlier that a prenatal exposure to a maternal high protein diet increased body fat by about 20–40% in adolescent and adult rats (Daenzer et al. 2002; Thone-Reineke et al. 2006). Increased energy intake in rodents can be caused by a higher dietary energy density usually due to a higher fat content either in a complete diet or in a cafeteria style diet designed to be highly palatable by the addition of sweet cream, cheese or chocolate bars to stimulate food intake (Vickers et al. 2000; Petry et al. 1997; Bayol et al. 2005). Rat offspring of mothers fed a high-fat diet during pregnancy have greater adiposity (Buckley et al. 2005b; Khan et al. 2003; Armitage et al. 2005). Feeding a cafeteria diet to pregnant and lactating rat dams resulted in markedly increased offspring adiposity at weaning (Bayol et al. 2005). In a model of obesity and glucose intolerance caused by hyperphagia (the gold thioglucose injected mouse) metabolic abnormalities are transferred to the next generation producing offspring which are also obese and glucose intolerant by 3 months of age (Buckley et al. 2005a).

3 Mechanisms

As indicated above there are differences between the maternal nutritional protocols causing imbalanced *in utero* or early postnatal nutrient supply associated with offspring adiposity. Thus, although tempting it is difficult to identify a common master regulator of programming effects in response to a variety of nutritional insults. Obesity is an energy balance problem and occurs when energy intake is too high in relation to energy output. Thus, one would expect alterations in components of energy balance such as energy expenditure/thermogenesis, food/energy intake, and locomotor activity in the programmed offspring. Among the several metabolic regulators underlying these components in the offspring, a closer look is given to the role of leptin and glucocorticoids.

3.1 Energy Expenditure, Food Intake, Physical Activity

To date there is only limited direct experimental evidence that there may be programming of components of energy balance in the offspring of mothers fed imbalanced diets during pregnancy. We observed reduced energy expenditure in 9 week old rat offspring prenatally exposed to a maternal high-protein diet which was associated with a higher body fat content (Daenzer et al. 2002). In mice offspring from undernourished (70% ad libitum intake) mothers, body fat was higher than in controls and energy expenditure was also reduced (Yura et al. 2005). Since energy expenditure measurements were not corrected for energy spent during physical activity in these reports, it remains to be elucidated if these reductions were due to decreased thermogenesis or physical activity level or both.

Food intake was reported to be programmed by either severe maternal UN or protein restriction during pregnancy (Vickers et al. 2000; Bellinger et al. 2006). In the study of Vickers and colleagues, increased food intake coincided with reduced physical activity and higher body fat, which resembles the so-called ‘couch-potato’ phenotype. Reduced locomotor activity in offspring during peripubertal and adult age was reported in a rat model of severe maternal UN during pregnancy and fed a hypercaloric diet after weaning (Vickers et al. 2003). Male offspring of pregnant rats restricted in dietary protein were less active than control animals which seemed to have no relation with body adiposity (Bellinger et al. 2006). Also in a rat model with a high intake of saturated fat during pregnancy a lower level of offspring locomotor activity was observed (Khan et al. 2003).

3.2 Leptin

Established obesity is characterized by high plasma concentrations of the adipocyte derived leptin reflecting the high body fat mass. Leptin is also produced in the placenta during pregnancy which is suspected to contribute to the increasing circulating levels

(Ashworth et al. 2000). Leptin increases energy expenditure, and modulates appetite by inhibition of hypothalamic arcuate nucleus (ARH) neurons producing neuropeptide Y and agouti-related peptide through the leptin receptor. In obese individuals, sustained elevated leptin levels are thought to cause selective leptin resistance at the hypothalamic level and thus leptin's anorectic action is blunted.

In rodents leptin levels are very low at birth but show a surge in release toward the end of the second postnatal week (Grove and Cowley 2005). The neonatal leptin surge occurs at a time when the ARH circuits are immature, and leptin is required for normal development of ARH pathways and later functioning of hypothalamic circuits that control feeding and energy expenditure (and thus adiposity). Mice neonates with fetal UN showed a premature onset of the neonatal leptin surge. A premature leptin surge generated by exogenous leptin administration in control offspring led to an accelerated weight gain with a high fat diet (Yura et al. 2005). However, injecting leptin into neonatal rat offspring of undernourished mothers prevents hyperphagia, and excessive body weight and fat mass gain (Vickers et al. 2005). These findings suggest that there is a role for leptin in hypothalamic programming of energy homeostasis. Thus, alterations of leptin levels during pre- to early postnatal key periods of hypothalamic development may programme selective leptin resistance and induce long-lasting effects on metabolism including an increased susceptibility to a postnatal obesogenic diet.

In contrast to neonatal rodents, less is known about the role of leptin in establishing hypothalamic feeding circuits in human babies. Serum leptin concentrations are high at birth but fall during the first days of life (Sarandakou et al. 2000). Small for gestational age newborns known to be at risk for becoming obese in later life had lower levels of cord leptin (Ong et al. 2000; Ong 2006). This suggests that leptin is also involved in the programming of energy balance in humans but it is important to consider species-related differences in development.

3.3 *Glucocorticoids*

Obesity is associated with increased cortisol production rate and increased 11ß-hydroxy-steroid dehydrogenase type 1 (11ßHSD1) mRNA and activity in adipose tissue while 11ß-HSD1 knockout mice are protected from obesity (reviewed in Walker 2007). Increased visceral adipose tissue glucocorticoid receptor (GR) concentration and local reactivation of cortisone to the active cortisol driven by 11ß-HSD1 plays a role in the pathophysiology of obesity. The biological activity of glucocorticoids is further determined by 11ß-hydroxy-steroid dehydrogenase type 2 (11ßHSD2) which inactivates active cortisol. Several lines of evidence suggest that glucocorticoids are implicated in the control of growth and the allocation of nutrients and energy in early life. Over the first 6 months of postnatal life GR and 11ßHSD1 mRNA abundance were positively related to adipose tissue weight in sheep (Gnanalingham et al. 2005). Rat overfeeding in the early postnatal period increased adipose tissue GR and 11ßHSD1 mRNA in adulthood (Boullo-Ciocca et al. 2005). In the MLP rat model a decreased placental 11ßHSD2 mRNA expression and activity was demonstrated implicating a cortisol overexposure of the fetus (Bertram et al. 2001; Stocker et al. 2004). When these pregnant rats were treated with leptin during the last trimester, placental 11ßHSD2 activity was unchanged and this was associated with less susceptibility to weight gain in the low birth weight rat offspring (Stocker et al. 2004). Maternal UN between early to mid gestation resulted in enhanced adipose tissue in neonatal sheep (Symonds et al. 2004), and was related to up-regulation of 11ßHSD1 and GR mRNA and a down-regulation of 11ßHSD2 in fetal peri-renal adipose tissue and at 6 months postnatal age (Gnanalingham et al. 2005). Further, chronic leptin injection reduces plasma cortisol levels and 11ßHSD2 mRNA but increases 11ßHSD1 and GR mRNA in sheep brown adipose tissue at 7 days postnatal age (Gnanalingham et al. 2005).

4 Conclusions

Many of the nutritional regimens used to model early life developmental programming of disease and obesity in rodent models are rather severe (e.g. Vickers et al. 2000). Nevertheless these models are useful to exhibit general principle mechanisms which might be partly active in humans. In conclusion, maternal imbalanced nutrition during pregnancy programmes systemic and adipose tissue glucocorticoid metabolism in the offspring by alteration of GR, 11ßHSD1 and 11ßHSD2 abundance and activity which may be modulated by leptin, suggesting a role in adipocyte metabolism and/or energy balance. Alterations of leptin levels during pre- and early postnatal key periods of hypothalamic development may programme selective leptin resistance and induce long-lasting metabolic effects. Variation of other determinant and possibly interacting factors such as ghrelin, insulin, triiodthyronin or uncoupling proteins may also be associated with nutritional programming of energy balance and obesity but which factor is cause and which effect is not, as yet, well understood.

References

Andreasyan, K., A.L. Ponsonby, T. Dwyer, R. Morley, M. Riley, K. Dear and J. Cochrane (2007). Higher maternal dietary protein intake in late pregnancy is associated with a lower infant ponderal index at birth. *Eur J Clin Nutr* **61**: 498–508.

Anguita, R.M., D.M. Sigulem and A.L. Sawaya (1993). Intrauterine food restriction is associated with obesity in young rats. *J Nutr* **123**: 1421–1428.

Armitage, J.A., I.Y. Khan, P.D. Taylor, P. Nathanielsz and L. Poston (2004). Developmental programming of the metabolic syndrome by maternal nutritional imbalance: how strong is the evidence from experimental models in mammals? *J Physiol* **561**(2): 355–377.

Armitage, J.A., P.D. Taylor and L. Poston (2005). Experimental models of developmental programming: consequences of exposure to an energy rich diet during development. *J Physiol* **565**(1): 3–8.

Ashworth, C.J., N. Hoggard, L. Thomas, J.G. Mercer, J.M. Wallace and R.G. Lea (2000). Placental leptin. *Rev Reprod* **5**: 18–24.

Bayol, S.A., B.H. Simbi and N.C. Stickland (2005). A maternal cafeteria diet during gestation and lactation promotes adiposity and impairs skeletal muscle development and metabolism in rat offspring at weaning. *J Physiol* **567**(Pt 3): 951–961.

Bellinger, L., D.V. Sculley and S.C. Langley-Evans (2006). Exposure to undernutrition in fetal life determines fat distribution, locomotor activity and food intake in ageing rats. *Int J Obes* **30**: 729–738.

Bertram, C., A.R. Trowern, N. Copin, A.A. Jackson and C.B. Whorwood (2001). The maternal diet during pregnancy programs altered expression of the glucocorticoid receptor and type 2 11beta-hydroxysteroid dehydrogenase: potential molecular mechanisms underlying the programming of hypertension *in utero*. *Endocrinology* **142**: 2841–2853.

Boney, C.M, A. Verma, R.Tucker and B.R. Vohr (2005). Metabolic syndrome in childhood: association with birth weight, maternal obesity, and gestational diabetes mellitus. *Pediatrics* **115**: e290–e296.

Boullo-Ciocca, S., A. Dutour, V. Guillaume, V. Achard, C. Oliver and M. Grino (2005). Postnatal diet-induced obesity in rats upregulates systemic and adipose tissue glucocorticoid metabolism during development and adulthood: its relationship with the metabolic syndrome. *Diabetologia* **54**: 197–203.

Buckley, A.J., A.L. Jaquiery and J.E. Harding (2005a). Nutritional programming of adult disease. *Cell Tissue Res* **322**: 73–79.

Buckley, A.J., B. Keseru, J. Briody, M. Thompson, S.E. Ozanne and C.H. Thompson (2005b). Altered body composition and metabolism in the male offspring of high fat-fed rats. *Metabolism* **54**: 500–507.

Cherala, G., B.H. Shapiro and A.P. D'mello (2006). Two low protein diets differentially affect food consumption in pregnant and lactating rats and long-term growth in their offspring. *J Nutr* **136**: 2827–2833.

Clancy, B., R.B. Darlington and B.L. Finlay (2001). Translating developmental time across mammalian species. *Neuroscience* **105**: 7–17.

Dörner, G. and A. Plagemann (1994). Perinatal hyperinsulinism as possible predisposing factor for diabetes mellitus, obesity and enhanced cardiovascular risk in later life. *Horm Metab Res* **26**: 213–21.

Daenzer, M., S. Ortmann, S. Klaus and C.C. Metges (2002). Prenatal high protein exposure decreases energy expenditure and increases adiposity in young rats. *J Nutr* **132**: 142–144.

Gluckman, P.D. and M.A. Hanson (2004). The developmental origins of the metabolic syndrome. *Trends Endocrinol Metab* **15**: 183–187.

Gnanalingham, M.G., A. Mostyn, M.E. Symonds and T. Stephenson (2005). Ontogeny and nutritional programming of adiposity in sheep: potential role of glucocorticoid action and uncoupling protein 2. *Am J Physiol Regul* **289**: 1407–1415.

Grove, K.L. and M.A. Cowley (2005). Is ghrelin a signal for the development of metabolic systems? *J Clin Invest* **115**: 3393–3397.

Hales, C.N. and D. J. Barker (1992). Type 2 (non-insulin-dependent) diabetes mellitus: the thrifty phenotype hypothesis. *Diabetologia* **35**: 595–601.

Keith, S.W., D.T. Redden, P.T. Katzmarzyk, M.M. Bogganio, E.C. Hanlon, R.M. Benca, D. Ruden, A. Pietrobelli, J.L. Barger, C. Wang et al. (2006). Putative contributors to the secular increase in obesity: exploring the roads less travelled. *Int J Obes* **30**: 1585–1594.

Kensara, O.A., S.A. Wootton, D.I. Phillips, M. Patel, A.A. Jackson and M. Elia (2005). Fetal programming of body composition: relation between birth weight and body composition measured by dual x-ray absorptiometry and anthropometric methods in older Englishmen. *Am J Clin Nutr* **82**: 980–987.

Khan, I.Y., P.D. Tylor, V. Dekou, P.T. Seed, L. Lakasing, D. Graham et al. (2003). Gender-linked hypertension in offspring of lard-fed pregnant rats. *Hypertension* **41**: 168–175.

Langley-Evans, S.C. (2000). Critical differences between two low protein diet protocols in the programming of hypertension in rats. *Int J Food Sci Nutr* **51**: 11–17.

Levin, B.E. and E. Govek (1998). Gestational obesity accentuates obesity in obesity-prone progeny. *Am J Physiol Regul* **275**: R1375–R1379.

Metges, C.C. and H.M. Hammon (2005). Nutritional programming: prenatal nutritional effects on the regulation of growth and metabolism. *J Anim Feed Sci* **14**(Suppl. 1): 15–30.

Okosun, I.S., Y. Liao, C.N. Rotimi, G.E. Dever and R.S. Cooper (2000). Impact of birth weight in ethnic variations in subcutaneous and central adiposity in American children aged 5–11 years. *Int J Obes Relat Metab Disord* **24**: 479–484.

Ong, K.K. (2006). Size at birth, postnatal growth and risk of obesity. *Horm Res* **65** (Suppl. 3): 65–69.
Ong, K.K., M.L. Ahmed, P.M. Emmett, M.A. Preece, D.B. Dunger and Avon Longitudinal study of pregnancy and childhood study team (2000). Association between postnatal catch-up growth and obesity in childhood: prospective cohort study. *Brit Med J* **320**: 967–971.
Owen, C.G., R.M. Martin, P.H. Whincup, G.D. Smith and D.G. Cook (2005). Effect of infant feeding on the risk of obesity across the life course: a quantitative review of published evidence. *Pediatrics* **115**: 1367–1377.
Ozaki, T., H. Nishina, A. Hanson and L. Poston (2001). Dietary restriction in pregnant rats causes gender-related hypertension and vascular dysfunction in offspring. *J Physiol* **530**: 141–152.
Ozanne, S.E. and C.N. Hales (2004). Lifespan: catch-up growth and obesity in male mice. *Nature* **427**(6973): 411–412.
Petry, C.J., S.E. Ozanne, C.L. Wang and C.N. Hales (1997). Early protein restriction and obesity independently induce hypertension in 1-year-old rats. *Clin Sci (Lond)* **93**: 147–152.
Sarandakou, A., E. Protonotariou, D. Rizos, A. Malamitsi-Puchner, G. Giannaki, I. Phocas and G. Creatsas (2000). Serum leptin concentrations during perinatal period. *Am J Perinatol* **17**: 325–328.
Stettler, N., V.A. Stallings, A.B. Troxel, J. Zhao, R. Schinnar, S.E. Nelson et al. (2005). Weight gain in the first week and life and overweight in adulthood: a cohort study of European American subjects fed infant formula. *Circulation* **111**: 1897–1903.
Stocker, C., J. O'Dowd, N.M. Morton, E. Wargent, M.V. Sennitt, D. Hislop, S. Glund, J.R. Seckl, J.R.S. Arch and M.A. Cawthorne (2004). Modulation of susceptibility to weight gain and insulin resistance in low birthweight rats by treatment of their mother with leptin during pregnancy and lactation. *Int J Obes* **28**: 129–136.
Symonds, M.E., A. Mostyn, S. Pearce, H. Budge and T. Stephenson (2003). Endocrine and nutritional regulation of fetal adipose tissue development. *J Endocrinol* **179**: 293–299.
Symonds, M.E., S. Pearce, J. Bispham, D.S. Gardner and T. Stephenson (2004). Timing of nutrient restriction and programming of fetal adipose tissue development. *Proc Nutr Soc* **63**: 397–403.
Thone-Reineke, C., P. Kalk, M. Dorn, S. Klaus, K. Simon, T. Pfab, M. Godes, P. Persson, T. Unger and B. Hocher (2006). High-protein nutrition during pregnancy and lactation programs blood pressure, food efficiency, and body weight of the offspring in a sex-dependent manner. *Am J Physiol Regul* **291**: R1025–R1030.
Vickers, M.H., B.H. Breier, W.S. Cutfield, P.L. Hofman and P.D. Gluckman (2000). Fetal origins of hyperphagia, obesity, and hypertension and postnatal amplification by hypercaloric nutrition. *Am J Physiol Endocrinol Metab* **279**: E83–E87.
Vickers, M.H., B.H. Breier, D. McCarthy and P.D. Gluckman (2003). Sedentary behaviour during postnatal life is determined by the prenatal environment and exacerbated by postnatal hypercaloric nutrition. *Am J Physiol Regul* **285**: R271–R273.
Vickers, M.H., P.D. Gluckman, A.H. Coveny, P.L. Hofman, W.S. Cutfield, A. Gertler, B.H. Breier and M. Harris (2005). Neonatal leptin treatment reverses developmental programming. *Endocrinology* **146**: 4211–4216.
Walker, B.R. (2007). Extra-adrenal regeneration of glucocorticoids by 11ß-hydroxysteroid dehydrogenase type 1: physiological regulator and pharmacological target for energy partitioning. *Proc Nutr Soc* **66**: 1–8.
Wallace, J.M., R.P. Aitken, J.S. Milne and W.W. Hay (2004). Nutritionally mediated placental growth restriction in the growing adolescent: consequences for the fetus. *Biol Reprod* **71**: 1055–1062.
Watson, R.E., J.M. DeSesso, M.E. Hurtt and G.D. Cappon (2006). Postnatal growth and morphological development of the brain: a species comparison. *Birth Def Res (Part B)* **77**: 471–484.
Westerterp-Platenga, M.S. (2003). The significance of protein in food intake and body weight regulation. *Curr Opin Clin Nutr Metab Care* **6**: 635–638.
Yura, S., H. Itoh, N. Sagawa, H. Yamamoto, H. Masuzaki, K. Nakao, M. Kawamura, M. Takemura, K. Kakui, Y. Ogawa and S. Fujii (2005). Role of premature leptin surge in obesity resulting from intrauterine undernutrition. *Cell Metab* **1**: 371–378.

Tissue Specific Adaptations to Nutrient Supply: More than Just Epigenetics?

Michael E. Symonds, Terence Stephenson, David S. Gardner, and Helen Budge

Abstract Changes in the maternal diet either throughout pregnancy, or at defined stages therein, can have pronounced effects on organogenesis in conjunction with endocrine sensitivity. These processes can be brought about by either maternal consumption of an imbalanced diet and/or a global reduction in macro or micronutrient intake. The magnitude of adaptation in the fetus or offspring is dependent on which organ is most rapidly growing and developing at that particular stage of the life cycle. For a majority of organs, the period of developmental plasticity extends beyond the fetal period, continuing through lactation and into the juvenile period. During lactation, enhanced growth of the offspring appears to be a primary determinant of the magnitude of adverse cardiovascular outcome. Consequently, a change in organ development during pregnancy may not necessarily equate with compromised function in later life. In the kidney, for example, adaptations in its endocrine sensitivity to maternal nutrient restriction through fetal development can be protective against the adverse consequences of later obesity. Such adaptations do not simply represent epigenetic modifications but a plethora of responses that, taken together, can prevent, or delay, at least in the kidney, the onset of apoptosis and later glomerulosclerosis.

Keywords Blood pressure • glucocorticoid receptor • kidney • obesity

Abbreviations AT_1: angiotensin-II receptor; GR: glucocorticoid receptor; IGF-I: insulin-like growth factor I; TNF: tumour necrosis factor; 11βHSD: 11β-hydroxysteroid dehydrogenase

---

M.E. Symonds (✉), T. Stephenson, D.S. Gardner, and H. Budge
Centre for Reproduction and Early Life, Institute of Clinical Research, University Hospital, Nottingham, NG7 2UH, UK
Michael.Symonds@nottingham.ac.uk

B. Koletzko et al. (eds.), *Early Nutrition Programming and Health Outcomes in Later Life: Obesity and Beyond*,

1 Introduction – Epigenetics and Development

Recent studies have indicated that pronounced changes in the maternal diet throughout pregnancy may be accompanied by epigenetic changes in the offspring (Waterland and Jirtle 2003), thereby providing one explanation for the long term nutritional programming of adult health and disease (Waterland and Jirtle 2004). To date, however, these types of studies have been based on very artificial conditions such as in vitro fertilization (Young et al. 2001) or have adopted a dietary composition that has little, if any, relationship to that consumed in the animals' natural environment (Waterland and Jirtle 2003; Waterland et al. 2006). The most widely quoted example of a dietary influence on epigenetics, as determined by variations in coat colour, relates to the effects of feeding mice a diet that contains extra folic acid, vitamin B12, choline, and betaine (Waterland and Jirtle 2003). This results in a marked change in coat colour with a shift from the yellow to the pseudo-agouti type. What must be noted with this model, however, is that only the latter coat colour is accompanied by a reduction in body weight and, thus, is a shift away from the obese phenotype (Dolinoy et al. 2006). It must, therefore, be emphasised that although nutritionally mediated mechanisms have been described with regard to the developmental regulation of coat colour in the mice (Waterland and Jirtle 2003), the same nutrients and mechanistic pathways may not explain the processes by which changes in micro and/or macronutrient intake during pregnancy and/or lactation impact on long term health and disease.

2 Ontogeny of Organ Development and Its Relationship with Endocrine Sensitivity

Another important consideration is the complexity of organ development and growth. In this regard, it is becoming clear that each organ has a pronounced specificity in its endocrine development that may relate, in part, to later function in both childhood and adult life (Gnanalingham et al. 2006). This is particularly notable with the glucocorticoid receptor (GR), for which an increase in abundance around the time of birth can be critical in determining effective adaptation to the extrauterine environment (Gnanalingham et al. 2005a, b). However, there are substantial differences in the maturity of organ development at birth between organs and between animal species at birth (Gnanalingham et al. 2005a, b). For example, in rats there is a pronounced plasticity in GR abundance in the kidney over the first 28 days of postnatal life which is profoundly influenced by the maternal diet during pregnancy (Brennan et al. 2008). A 50% reduction in maternal food intake significantly increases GR abundance at 7 days after birth but, interestingly, not between 14 and 28 days. As adults, these offspring show increased renal GR protein with a reduction in nephron number but, perhaps surprisingly, have lower, rather than elevated, blood pressure when measured by telemetry over a 24 h period (Brennan et al. 2006, 2008).

One major factor that appears to determine the magnitude of adverse adaptation in rat offspring following maternal nutritional manipulation through pregnancy is the time at which the diet is restored to that of controls (Symonds 2007). This in turn is related to the degree of accelerated whole body growth rate after birth. Consequently, when the mother is maintained on a low-protein high-carbohydrate through lactation and the offspring are then weaned onto the same diet, they remain smaller than offspring born to control fed dams and show both a reduction in nephron number as well as lower resting blood pressure (Hoppe et al. 2007).

3 Maternal Nutrient Restriction Coincident with the Period of Placental Growth and Its Impact on the Kidney Following Obesity

We have previously established that, in sheep, maternal nutrient restriction targeted from the period in which uterine attachment occurs i.e. ~28 days gestation up to the period at which placental weight is maximal i.e. 80 days gestation results in a reduction in the mean weight of individual placentomes (Clarke et al. 1998; Heasman et al. 1998). This occurs in conjunction with a reduced potential capacity to inactivate maternal cortisol through the enzyme 11β-hydroxysteroid dehydrogenase (11βHSD) type 2 (Whorwood et al. 2001) which may be in response to a decrease in maternal plasma cortisol (Bispham et al. 2003). It also is the period in which fetal nephrogenesis occurs (Wintour and Moritz 1997). At term, the offspring have larger kidneys, surrounded by more adipose tissue (Bispham et al. 2003) than controls and in which there is increased mRNA abundance for the GR in adipose tissue and the glucocorticoid responsive angiotensin-II receptor (AT_1) in the kidney (Whorwood et al. 2001).

As juveniles, resting blood pressure is reduced in offspring born to nutrient restricted mothers when their fat mass is unaffected (Gopalakrishnan et al. 2005). In view of these results, we have recently investigated the impact of a post weaning obesogenic environment on the long term outcomes. To our surprise, offspring born to nutrient restricted mothers showed no differences in their enhanced fat mass compared with controls or in the effects of obesity on either increased blood pressure or altered kidney function. However, despite there being a similar increase in fat mass around the kidney between obese and nutrient restricted obese offspring, we observed pronounced differences in renal adaptations in response to obesity. In this regard, there was significant cortical apoptosis and glomerulosclerosis in conjunction with upregulation of mRNA for the GR, AT_1R and tumour necrosis factor (TNF)-α within the kidneys of obese animals compared with age-matched lean offspring that was not seen in the obese nutrient restricted group (Williams et al. 2007). These unique findings, therefore, suggest that nutrient restriction *in utero* that is targeted specifically during the period in which nephrogenesis occurs confers apparent renal protection from some of the tissue structural effects of obesity. In the obese controls, increased renal expression of GR, TNF-α and AT_1, indicate the potential for enhanced cortisol sensitivity, local pro-inflammatory cytokine activity and local vasoconstriction, respectively. Prenatal nutrient restriction prevented all local molecular changes and any signs of regional apoptosis or glomerulosclerosis for which epigenetic modification does not provide an obvious mechanism. One explanation as to why the kidneys of offspring born to nutrient restricted mothers are less susceptible to apoptosis may be related to increased IGF-I receptor abundance (Brennan et al. 2005) that would be predicted to promote cell survival (Rajah et al. 1997) rather than apoptosis.

These results are potentially applicable to the human situation since the magnitude of maternal nutritional manipulation we have utilised is comparable to contemporary populations in which a 50% variation in maternal food intake between the upper and lower quartiles is apparent during pregnancy (Godfrey et al. 1996). In addition, for many women a comparative nutrient restriction occurs in early to mid gestation due to the accompanying nausea suffered by nearly 90% of pregnant women in the UK. Indeed, nausea in pregnancy has been suggested to be closely associated with the maternal diet in Western women (Pepper and Roberts 2006).

4 Conclusion

In summary, epigenetic mechanisms appear to be only one explanation as to how fetal growth and organ development can be reset following physiological changes in the maternal diet. Given the current concern that there may be transgenerational responses following increased exposure to such nutrients as folic acid (Lucock and Yates 2005), much more detailed studies in a range of experimental animal models are required in order to ascertain whether widespread dietary fortification is a wise strategy for improving the health of the population.

Acknowledgements The work was supported by a British Heart Foundation and the European Union Sixth Framework Programme for Research and Technical Development of the European Community – The Early Nutrition Programming Project (FOOD-CT-2005-007036).

References

Bispham, J., G. S. Gopalakrishnan, J. Dandrea, V. Wilson, H. Budge, D. H. Keisler, F. Broughton Pipkin, T. Stephenson and M. E. Symonds (2003). "Maternal endocrine adaptation throughout pregnancy to nutritional manipulation: consequences for maternal plasma leptin and cortisol and the programming of fetal adipose tissue development." *Endocrinology* **144**: 3575–3585.

Brennan, K. A., G. S. Gopalakrishnan, L. Kurlak, S. M. Rhind, C. E. Kyle, A. N. Brooks, M. T. Rae, D. M. Olson, T. Stephenson and M. E. Symonds (2005). "Impact of maternal undernutrition and fetal number on glucocorticoid, growth hormone and insulin-like growth factor receptor mRNA abundance in the ovine fetal kidney." *Reproduction* **129**(2): 151–159.

Brennan, K. A., D. M. Olson and M. E. Symonds (2006). "Maternal nutrient restriction alters renal development and blood pressure regulation of the offspring." *Proc Nutr Soc* **65**(1): 116–124.

Brennan, K. A., S. Kaufman, S. W. Reynolds, B. T. McCook, G. Kan, I. Christiaens, M. E. Symonds and D. Olson (2008). "Differential the effects of maternal nutrient restriction through pregnancy

on kidney development and later blood pressure control in the resulting offspring." *Am J Physiol* 295, R197–R205.
Clarke, L., L. Heasman, D. T. Juniper and M. E. Symonds (1998). "Maternal nutrition in early-mid gestation and placental size in sheep." *Brit J Nutr* **79**: 359–364.
Dolinoy, D. C., J. R. Weidman, R. A. Waterland and R. L. Jirtle (2006). "Maternal genistein alters coat color and protects Avy mouse offspring from obesity by modifying the fetal epigenome." *Environ Health Perspect* **114**(4): 567–572.
Gnanalingham, M. G., A. Mostyn, J. Dandrea, D. P. Yakubu, M. E. Symonds and T. Stephenson (2005a). "Ontogeny and nutritional programming of uncoupling protein-2 and glucocorticoid receptor mRNA in the ovine lung." *J Physiol (Lond)* **565**: 159–169.
Gnanalingham, M. G., A. Mostyn, M. E. Symonds and T. Stephenson (2005b). "Ontogeny and nutritional programming of adiposity: potential role of glucocorticoid sensitivity and uncoupling protein-2." *Am J Physiol* **289**: R1407–R1415.
Gnanalingham, M. G., A. Mostyn, D. S. Gardner, T. Stephenson and M. E. Symonds (2006). "Developmental regulation of the lung in preparation for life after birth: nutritional manipulation of local glucocorticoid action and uncoupling protein 2." *J Endocrinol* **188**: 375–386.
Godfrey, K., S. Robinson, D. J. P. Barker, C. Osmond and V. Cox (1996). "Maternal nutrition in early and late pregnancy in relation to placental and fetal growth." *BMJ* **312**: 410–414.
Gopalakrishnan, G., D. S. Gardner, J. Dandrea, S. C. Langley-Evans, S. Pearce, L. O. Kurlak, R. M. Walker, I. Sweetho, D. H. Keisler, M. M. Ramsay, T. Stephenson and M. E. Symonds (2005). "Influence of maternal pre-pregnancy body composition and diet during early-mid pregnancy on cardiovascular function and nephron number in juvenile sheep." *Brit J Nutr* **94**: 938–947.
Heasman, L., L. Clarke, K. Firth, T. Stephenson and M. E. Symonds (1998). "Influence of restricted maternal nutrition in early to mid gestation on placental and fetal development at term in sheep." *Pediatr Res* **44**: 546–551.
Hoppe, C. C., R. G. Evans, K. M. Moritz, L. A. Cullen-McEwen, S. M. Fitzgerald, J. Dowling and J. F. Bertram (2007). "Combined prenatal and postnatal protein restriction influences adult kidney structure, function, and arterial pressure." *Am J Physiol* **292**(1): R462–R469.
Lucock, M. and Z. Yates (2005). "Folic acid – vitamin and panacea or genetic time bomb?" *Nat Rev Genet* **6**(3): 235–240.
Pepper, G. and S. Roberts (2006). "Rates of nausea and vomiting in pregnancy and dietary characteristics across populations." *Proc R Soc Biol Sci* **273**: 2675–2679.
Rajah, R., B. Valentinis and P. Cohen (1997). "Insulin-like growth factor (IGF)-binding protein-3 induces apoptosis and mediates the effects of transforming growth factor-beta1 on programmed cell death through a p53- and IGF-independent mechanism." *J Biol Chem* **272**(18): 12181–12188.
Symonds, M. E. (2007). "Integration of physiological and molecular mechanisms of the developmental origins of adult disease: new concepts and insights." *Proc Nutr Soc* **66**: 442–450.
Waterland, R. A. and R. L. Jirtle (2003). "Transposable elements: targets for early nutritional effects on epigenetic gene regulation." *Mol Cell Biol* **23**: 5293–5300.
Waterland, R. A. and R. L. Jirtle (2004). "Early nutrition, epigenetic changes at transposons and imprinted genes, and enhanced susceptibility to adult chronic diseases." *Nutrition* **20**(1): 63–68.
Waterland, R. A., J. R. Lin, C. A. Smith and R. L. Jirtle (2006). "Post-weaning diet affects genomic imprinting at the insulin-like growth factor 2 (Igf2) locus." *Hum Mol Genet* **15**(5): 705–716.
Whorwood, C. B., K. M. Firth, H. Budge and M. E. Symonds (2001). "Maternal undernutrition during early- to mid-gestation programmes tissue-specific alterations in the expression of the glucocorticoid receptor, 11β-hydroxysteroid dehydrogenase isoforms and type 1 angiotensin II receptor in neonatal sheep." *Endocrinology* **142**: 2854–2864.
Williams, P., L. O. Kurlak, A. Perkins, H. Budge, T. Stephenson, D. H. Keisler, M. E. Symonds and D. S. Gardner (2007). "Impaired renal function and hypertension accompany juvenile obesity: effect of prenatal diet." *Kidney Int* **72**(3): 279–289, doi: 10.1038/sj.ki5002276.

Wintour, E. M. and K. M. Moritz (1997). "Comparative aspects of fetal renal development." *Equine Vet J* **24**: 51–58.

Young, L., K. Fernandes, T. McEvoy, S. Butterwith, C. Gutierrez, C. Carolan, P. Broadbent, J. Robinson, I. Wilmut and K. Sinclair (2001). "Epigenetic change in IGF2R is associated with fetal overgrowth after embryo culture." *Nat Genet* **27**: 153–154.

Epigenetics – Potential Contribution to Fetal Programming

John C. Mathers and Jill A. McKay

Abstract Whilst the primary DNA sequence sets the limits of potential gene expression, the pattern of gene expression in a given cell under particular circumstances is determined by several factors including the epigenetic marking of the genome. These marks include DNA methylation and post-translational modification of the histones around which DNA is wrapped when packaged in the nucleus. Importantly, these marks are malleable in response to environmental exposures and contribute to phenotypic plasticity in the context of a fixed genotype. There is now proof of principle that maternal diet can have a profound impact on the epigenome and so determine gene expression patterns and health throughout the life-course. Studies of altered epigenetic marking will be of profound importance for mechanistic understanding of the role of nutrition in health but especially for studies of the developmental origins of health.

Keywords DNA methylation • epigenetics • gene expression • histone decoration

Abbreviations GR: glucocorticoid receptor; IGF2: insulin-like growth factor 2; PPARα: peroxisome proliferator-activated receptor alpha; PR: protein-restricted

1 Environmental Signals

Biennial plants, such as members of the Brassica family, flower only after exposure to an extended cold period (winter), a process known as vernalisation. In these cases, the signalling for the initial stages of sexual reproduction involves the Flowering Locus C (FLC) protein which represses expression of genes needed for flowering.

J.C. Mathers
Human Nutrition Research Centre, School of Clinical Medical Sciences, Newcastle University, William Leech Building, Framlington Place, Newcastle on Tyne, NE2 4HH, UK
john.mathers@newcastle.ac.uk

B. Koletzko et al. (eds.), *Early Nutrition Programming and Health Outcomes in Later Life: Obesity and Beyond,*

Vernalisation includes down-regulation of *FLC* expression (Bastow et al. 2004). This change in gene expression, with profound implications for plant function, is determined by epigenetic mechanisms. Bastow et al. (2004) conclude that 'the epigenetic memory of winter is mediated by a "histone code" that specifies a silent chromatin state conserved between animals and plants'. Evidence is now accumulating that a variety of environmental signals, including nutrition, influences mammalian function and health through epigenetic mechanisms (Jirtle and Skinner 2007).

2 Epigenetic Mechanisms

The primary DNA sequence of any genome defines the potential for gene expression. However, superimposed on the primary (genetic) sequence is an information-rich epigenetic layer which has a major influence on what genes are expressed in a specific cell at a given moment in time. Epigenetics describes genomic markings (chemical modifications) which are heritable from one cell generation to the next but do not involve changes in the primary DNA sequence (Bernstein et al. 2007). The best known epigenetic marks are (i) methylation of cytosines in CpG dinucleotides and (ii) post-translational modifications of histones. The epigenome refers to the totality of epigenetic marks in a given cell under particular circumstances. Together these chemical modifications regulate chromatin structure and accessibility to DNA of the transcriptional machinery. At its simplest, methylation of CpG rich regions (CpG islands) in promoters acts to switch off the associated gene. These discoveries have led to the hypothesis that epigenetics is a key mechanism allowing phenotypic plasticity in the context of a fixed genotype. Unlike DNA mutations which can also alter cellular phenotype e.g. in a tumour cell, epigenetic markings are potentially reversible. Further, since epigenetic marks can be modified by environmental factors, the epigenome is a means to connect environmental exposure with gene expression and cell/tissue function. This may be especially important for early life (*in utero*) exposures. In the very earliest stages of life the genome undergoes radical changes in epigenetic marks which are characterised by waves of de-methylation of DNA followed by re-methylation (Reik et al. 2001). Since epigenetic markings are propagated through mitosis in somatic cells, aberrant marks may have consequences for gene expression in all tissues throughout the life course. These epigenetic mechanisms may provide (at least in part) a mechanistic explanation for the observations that a wide range of prenatal and early postnatal exposures (including dietary components, xenobiotic chemicals, behavioural cues and low-dose radiation) influence disease risk in later life (Jirtle and Skinner 2007).

3 The Four "Rs" of Epigenomics

The mechanistic connection between environmental exposures and altered health through epigenetic processes includes several key stages which we have termed *the four* "**R**s" *of epigenomics*. This encapsulates the processes involved in (i) **R**eceiving environmental signals, (ii) **R**ecording that environmental exposure through altered patterns of epigenomic marks, (iii) **R**emembering the resulting epigenomic pattern through subsequent cell divisions and (iv) **R**evealing the consequences of the altered epigenomic markings in the cell's unique transcriptome. There is a good working model for the process by which DNA methylation marks are copied during mitosis (**R**emembering). The "maintenance" DNA methyltransferase (DNMT1) catalyses methylation (S-adenosyl methionine is the methyl donor) of CpGs in the newly synthesised DNA (daughter) strand using the pattern of cytosine methylation marks in the template (parental) strand (Bird 2002). In contrast, there is limited understanding of the other three "**R**s". In particular, little is known about the epigenetic targets of environmental exposures which will lead to differential gene expression. Jirtle and Skinner (2007) suggest that these are likely to include (i) the promoter regions of house-keeping genes (well-described for numerous tumour suppressor genes), (ii) genes with metastable epialleles i.e. loci that can be epigenetically modified in a variable (and reversible) manner to give a distribution of phenotypes from genetically identical cells and (iii) imprinted genes, i.e. genes that are expressed in a parent-of-origin specific manner e.g. that for insulin-like growth factor 2 (*IGF2*) is normally expressed only from the allele inherited from the father (in humans and mice).

4 Fetal Exposures and the Epigenome

Supplementation of the maternal diet of viable yellow agouti (A^{vy}) mice with methyl donors (folic acid, vitamin B12, choline and betaine) alters the phenotype of the offspring and results in a higher proportion of pups with brown (pseudo-agouti) rather than yellow or mottled coats (Waterland and Jirtle 2003). This shift in coat colour is due to increased methylation of CpGs upstream of a transposable element which alters expression of the *agouti* gene (Waterland and Jirtle 2003). In the same mouse model, supplementing the maternal diet with 250 mg genistein/kg from 2 weeks before mating has a similar effect on coat colour and is associated with increased methylation of six CpGs in the retrotransposon upstream of the transcription start site for the *agouti* gene (Dolinoy et al. 2006). Interestingly, there was less obesity in the offspring of the genistein-supplemented dams (Dolinoy et al. 2006). The extent of methylation of these CpG dinucleotides was similar in tissues derived from different embryonic cell lineages and was unaltered by age of mouse suggesting that genistein exposure alters methylation profiles ***before*** embryonic stem cell differentiation and so produces permanent changes in the epigenome (Dolinoy et al. 2006).

It is now well-established that feeding protein-restricted (PR) diets to pregnant rats induces offspring phenotypes which have characteristics of the metabolic syndrome e.g. raised blood pressure (Bertram and Hanson 2001). Such offspring have hypomethylation of the promoters, and increased expression, of the peroxisome proliferator-activated receptor (*PPAR*)α and glucocorticoid receptor (*GR*) genes in liver of recently-weaned offspring (Lillycrop et al. 2005). High-dose supplementation of the PR diet with folic acid reversed these changes (Lillycrop et al. 2005).

Changes in epigenetic markings as a result of environmental (dietary) exposures are not restricted to the early stages of life. In a ground-breaking study of monozygotic twins, Fraga et al. (2005) demonstrated that epigenomic markings (chromosomal patterns of DNA methylation) diverged as twins aged and that this was accompanied by greater inter-twin differences in gene expression. Some discordance in epigenetic markings with age would be expected because of stochastic (i.e. random) events e.g. during mitosis, copying of DNA methylation marks is much less well policed than is copying of the primary genetic sequence. However, the extent of discordance in both DNA methylation patterns and in gene expression in the study by Fraga et al. (2005) was greater for those twin pairs who had lived more of their lives apart suggesting that environmental factors may play an important role in determining not only epigenomic characteristics but also disease risk (Poulsen et al. 2007). The mechanisms through which (maternal or post-weaning) dietary factors modulate epigenetic markings remain poorly understood.

5 Summary and Working Hypotheses

In summary, it is becoming evident that altered epigenetic marking is:

- A means through which evidence of environmental exposures is **R**eceived and **R**ecorded by the genome
- **R**emembered through multiple cell generations
- **R**evealed in altered gene expression (and cell function) and
- Observed during disease development and in ageing

It seems likely that studies of altered epigenetic marking will be of profound importance for mechanistic understanding of the role of nutrition in health but especially for studies of the developmental origins of health because altered epigenetic marking:

- Allows plasticity of phenotype in a fixed genotype
- Is implicated in the aetiology of many diseases and may be causal for some
- Connects environmental exposure with gene expression and function
- *Appears* to be modifiable by nutritional intervention and
- May be more sensitive to diet during early development

Acknowledgements Research in my laboratory on early nutrition, epigenetics and health is funded by the Biotechnology and Biological Sciences Research Council through the Centre for Integrated Systems Biology of Ageing and Nutrition (CISBAN) (BB/C008200/1) and through the Focus Team on "Nutritional Epigenomics" within NuGO 'The European Nutrigenomics Organisation; linking genomics, nutrition and health research' (CT-2004-505944) an EU FP6 Network of Excellence.

References

Bastow, R., J.S. Mylne, C. Lister, Z. Lippman, R.A. Martienssen and C. Dean (2004) "Vernalization requires epigenetic silencing of *FLC* by histone methylation." *Nature* **427**: 164–167.

Bernstein, B.E., A. Meissner and E.S. Lander (2007) "The mammalian epigenome." *Cell* **128**: 669–681.

Bertram, C.E. and M.A. Hanson (2001) "Animal models and programming of the metabolic syndrome." *Brit Med Bull* **60**: 103–121.

Bird, A. (2002) "DNA methylation patterns and epigenetic memory." *Genes Dev* **16**: 6–21.

Dolinoy, D.C., J.R. Weidman, R.A. Waterland and R.L. Jirtle (2006) "Maternal genistein alters coat colour and protects Avy mouse offspring from obesity by modifying the fetal epigenome." *Environ Health Perspect* **114**(4): 567–572.

Fraga, M.F., E. Ballestar, M.F. Paz, S. Ropero, F. Setien, M.L. Ballestar, D. Heine-Suner, J.C. Cigudosa, M. Urioste, J. Benitez, M. Boix-Chornet, A. Sanchez-Aguilera, C. Ling, E. Carlsson, P. Poulsen, A. Vaag, Z. Stephan, T.D. Spector, Y.Z. Wu, C. Plass and M. Esteller (2005) "Epigenetic differences arise during the lifetime of monozygotic twins." *Proc Natl Acad Sci USA* **102**(30): 10604–10609.

Jirtle, R.L. and M.K. Skinner (2007) "Environmental epigenomics and disease susceptibility." *Nat Rev Genet* **8**: 253–262.

Lillycrop, K.A., E.S. Phillips, A.A. Jackson, M.A. Hanson and G.C. Burdge (2005) "Dietary restriction of pregnant rats induces and folic acid supplementation prevents epigenetic modification of hepatic gene expression in the offspring." *J Nutr* **135**: 1382–1386.

Poulsen, P., M. Esteller, A. Vaag and M.F. Fraga (2007) "The epigenetic basis of twin discordance in age-related diseases." *Pediatr Res* **61**(5): 38R–42R.

Reik, W., W. Dean and J. Walter (2001) "Epigenetic reprogramming in mammalian development." *Science* **293**: 1089–1093.

Waterland, R.A. and R.L. Jirtle (2003) "Transposable elements: targets for early nutritional effects on epigenetic gene regulation." *Mol Cell Biol* **23**: 5293–5300.

Programming of Impaired Insulin Secretion Versus Sensitivity: Cause or Effect?

Brigitte Reusens and Claude Remacle

Abstract A substantial body of evidence suggests that a poor intrauterine milieu elicited by maternal nutritional disturbance, including maternal diabetes or placental insufficiency, may programme susceptibility in the fetus to later development of glucose intolerance and diabetes. Numerous data in animals have allowed possible mechanisms for programming to be proposed. This review of work in several animal models attempts to identify the cellular and molecular mechanisms at the level of the beta-cell and in the insulin sensitive tissues that are involved in the process of events leading to the pathology later in life.

Keywords Animal models • beta cell • diabetes • early programming • insulin target tissues

Abbreviations IGF: insulin like growth factor; IUGR: intrauterine growth retardation; VEGF: vascular endothelial growth factor

1 Poor Fetal Growth and Risk of Glucose Intolerance and Diabetes in Later Life in Humans

An association has been found between fetal and infant growth and subsequent impaired glucose tolerance and type 2 diabetes in elderly men (Hales et al. 1991). The relation may be U-shaped or reversed J-shaped (Rich-Edwards et al. 1999). Studies of individuals exposed *in utero* to famine during the Dutch Hunger Winter in 1944–1945 have shown directly that maternal malnutrition, especially during the last trimester of pregnancy, led to growth restriction of the fetus and was associated with

B. Reusens(✉) and C. Remacle(✉)
Laboratoire de Biologie Cellulaire, Institut des Sciences de la Vie,
Université catholique de Louvain, 5 place Croix du Sud, 1348 Louvain-la-Neuve, Belgique
reusens@bani.ucl.ac.be, remacle@bani.ucl.ac.be

B. Koletzko et al. (eds.), *Early Nutrition Programming and Health Outcomes in Later Life: Obesity and Beyond*,

impaired glucose tolerance and insulin resistance in 50-year old offspring (Ravelli et al. 1998). There was also a negative relationship with birth weight and the risk of gestational diabetes (Innes et al. 2002). In addition, risk factors for insulin resistance, type-2 diabetes and obesity were also conveyed by intrauterine exposure to diabetes which affects fetal organ development and more specifically the endocrine pancreas (Van Assche et al. 1977). Indeed, offspring from mothers with diabetes (type 1 and type 2) featured altered beta-cell function as assessed by higher insulin content in the amniotic fluid. Molsted-Pedersen et al. (1972) proposed that increased fetal insulin secretion and consequently fetal growth resulted from a combination of higher maternal glucose, amino acids and lipids crossing the placenta. In the Pima Indian population, in which diabetes has the highest prevalence in the world, the risk of diabetes was higher in siblings born from diabetic mothers than in those born before the mother became diabetic (Dabelea et al. 2000) which further points towards a detrimental effect of gestational diabetes on the health of the offspring.

2 Type 2 Diabetes

Type 2 diabetes is characterized by four major metabolic abnormalities which are obesity, impaired insulin action, insulin secretion dysfunction and increased endogenous glucose output (Leahy 2005). It is clear that the three first anomalies are already present in most individuals long before the onset of the disease, but what is unclear is the sequence in which they develop, as well as their relative contribution to the progressive development of glucose intolerance and later to frank diabetes, but the fetal environment has been demonstrated to take part in these processes.

To attempt to delineate this sequence of events and to understand the mechanisms that underlie the early programming of glucose intolerance and type 2 diabetes, many animal models have been used, some of them having provided some useful information. Different modes of malnutrition occurring during different periods of development have been set up: calorie or protein restriction, uterine artery ligation, gestational diabetes and high fat diet. In each model, alterations in the development of several organs were observed and later consequences for the health of the progeny were reported. Abundant literature demonstrates the unambiguous role of the intrauterine metabolic environment on the insulin target tissues and the occurrence of impaired insulin secretion, glucose intolerance and diabetes later in life. Data on the effect on fetal beta-cell development are less numerous but they are also clear. However, a question remains: what comes first in the programming sequence? Is it the beta-cells or the insulin-sensitive targeted tissues which are programmed first?

3 Programming of the Beta-Cells

The development of the endocrine pancreas follows a similar pattern in all mammals, but the sequence of events may vary from one species to another which could be important when nutritional perturbation occurs since critical windows exist. In rat, the development of the endocrine pancreas starts from a pool of common precursor cells that become progressively committed to the endocrine lineage under the control of a hierarchical network of transcription factors. At birth, the beta-cell mass is determined by the recruitment of undifferentiated precursors, as well as the replication and apoptosis rates of the beta-cells. Obviously, any disturbance of the environment of the endocrine cells at a specific developmental time point, may perturb the balance of controlling factors, thereby contributing to beta-cell abnormalities and diabetes later in life.

3.1 Models of Undernutrition

The size of the beta-cell mass depends on whether the fetus grows in a restricted or an abundant nutritional environment. Fetuses exposed to a low protein diet during gestation or to 50% calorie intake from the last week of gestation exhibited a lower beta-cell mass at birth. (Snoeck et al. 1990; Garofano et al. 1997). The mass of the endocrine pancreas was reduced by approximately 30% in the malnourished offspring in both models compared to the controls. The mechanisms leading to the defective development, however, are thought to be different. In the fetuses from the maternal low-protein model, the replication rate of beta-cells was diminished by about 50% and the apoptotic rate was increased (Petrik et al. 1999). The fetuses not only had fewer beta-cells but their islets were poorly vascularised (Snoeck et al. 1990; Boujendar et al. 2003) and secreted less insulin in response to amino acids (Cherif et al. 2001). Factors such as a lower level of insulin-like growth factor (IGF), vascular endothelial growth factor (VEGF) (Boujendar et al. 2003) and taurine may play a role in the underdevelopment of the beta-cell mass. In contrast, in the fetuses from the low-calorie diet model, the lower beta-cell mass was not attributed to reduced proliferation or increased apoptosis, but rather to an alteration in islet neogenesis (Garofano et al. 1997). In this model, the role of the high level of glucocorticoids seems determinant for the low beta-cell mass (Blondeau et al. 2001).

Intrauterine growth retardation can also be mimicked in animals by ligation of the uterine artery on the last days of gestation (Boloker et al. 2002). Although no difference in the beta-cell mass was detected at 1 and 7 weeks, growth retarded pups exhibited a reduced beta-cell proliferation at 14 days postnatally but a normal apoptotic rate. The level of pancreatic and duodenal homeobox 1 (Pdx1) mRNA was dramatically decreased in the fetal beta-cell and the reduced expression persisted after birth until 3 months.

3.2 Models of Overnutrition

As well as undernutrition, studies have shown that overnutrition during fetal life can also lead to increased risk of diabetes in adulthood. In rats, diabetes may be induced experimentally by streptozotocin injection, which selectively destroys beta-cells and mild or severe diabetes ensues depending on the dose used. At birth, the progeny of mild diabetic dams were macrosomic (i.e. large for gestational age) and the development of the endocrine pancreas was enhanced by increased blood glucose concentration resulting in an enhanced volume of endocrine tissue due to hyperplasia and hypertrophy of the islets of Langerhans (Aerts and Van Assche 2006). Islet cell proliferation was increased by 42%, leading to higher beta-cell mass that was hyper-vascularized (Reusens and Remacle 2001). A high fat diet from weaning until adulthood and throughout gestation also affected the development of the endocrine pancreas of the fetus (Srinivasan et al. 2006). Taken together all these data show that early metabolic disturbance alters the development of the endocrine pancreas by influencing the differentiation or the proliferation of the beta-cells with consequences existing already at birth.

4 Programming of the Insulin Sensitive Target Tissues

4.1 Models of Undernutrition

The poor development of the endocrine pancreas after early malnutrition leaves the offspring with a sub-optimal complement of functional units. However, the exhaustion of the low beta-cell mass generated early in life may only be clearly revealed in situations of increased insulin demand such as obesity, pregnancy or aging. Islets from 3 month-old adult offspring from dams exposed to a low protein diet during gestation released less insulin when stimulated *in vitro* with glucose or amino acids (Dahri et al. 1991). A lower insulin secretion was apparent *in vivo* after an oral glucose test in 3 month-old offspring from mother fed the low calorie or the low protein diet during gestation and lactation (Garofano et al. 1998; Merezak et al. 2004) although no glucose intolerance was detected at that age. However they underwent a greater age dependent loss of glucose tolerance than control offspring and developed impaired glucose tolerance at 15 months (Ozanne et al. 2003) and frank diabetes by 17 months of age (Petry et al. 2001). The impact of maternal low protein diet on insulin sensitivity paralleled the changes observed in glucose tolerance. Improved whole body, muscle and adipose tissue insulin sensitivity was observed in young adult life. However in old age, insulin resistance was reported (Ozanne et al. 2003). This was associated with changes in the expression of key insulin signalling molecules such as the p110 beta subunit of phosphatidylinositol (PI) 3-kinase in adipose tissue and protein kinase C zeta in muscle (Ozanne et al. 2001). Interestingly, similar changes in the expression of these insulin signalling proteins were observed in muscle biopsies from low birth weight men (Ozanne et al. 2005).

A drastic 70% reduction of food intake during gestation in rats induced a growth retardation at birth. At 100 days the restricted offspring exhibited a higher plasma insulin level which was exacerbated by a high fat diet postnatally (Vickers et al. 2000).

The offspring of mothers with bilateral uterine artery ligation the last 3 days of gestation were intrauterine growth retarded (IUGR). At 7 weeks, these offspring were glucose intolerant and insulin resistant as revealed by an intravenous glucose tolerance test. At 15 months, they were unable to secrete insulin in response to the same challenge.

4.2 Models of Overnutrition

An abundance of nutrients during gestation and lactation also compromises the insulin sensitivity in the adult progeny. Indeed in rats, diabetes during pregnancy may convey glucose intolerance in the adult offspring that become insulin deficient or insulin resistant depending on the severity of the maternal hyperglycemia (Aerts and Van Assche 2006). In addition, adult offspring from dams fed on a high fat diet during gestation and lactation, featured an hyperinsulinemia and a decreased insulin sensitivity even though they had islets containing less insulin and that secreted less insulin *in vitro* in response to glucose (Taylor et al. 2005).

4.3 A Common Mechanism?

A common mechanism by which all the disparate intrauterine insults proceed to exert an effect on the insulin sensitive tissues in the offspring may be via mitochondrial programming. It has been proposed that a limited or an excess of energy in the early environment may reprogram mitochondrial function in different organs (Peterside et al. 2003; Taylor et al. 2005). The beta-cell has a higher energy requirement and a lower antioxidant defence than many other tissues (Tiedge et al. 1997). It thus may be a susceptible target for mitochondrial reprogramming which will lead to increased reactive oxygen species (ROS) production, which in turn will damage the mitochondrial DNA (Simmons et al. 2005). The proteome analysis of islets from fetuses of mothers fed a low protein diet revealed that the expression of proteins involved in the mitochondrial energy transfer, glucose metabolism, RNA and DNA metabolism was changed compared to normal progeny (Sparre et al. 2003).

5 Conclusions

Animal studies have offered data that shed some light on the mechanisms leading to glucose intolerance and insulin resistance when the intrauterine environment was disturbed. They have helped to show that early alteration in the development of the beta- cells leads to disturbed beta-cell function. Insulin sensitive tissues appear to adapt by increasing insulin sensitivity but with obesity, pregnancy or aging, insulin resistance appears and type 2 diabetes may ensue. These data would suggest that it is the beta-cells which are programmed first.

Does such a sequence of events reflect the human situation? It is not possible to answer this question, although recently attention was paid to the beta-cell mass in humans (Butler et al. 2003). Pancreases from lean and obese persons with normal glucose levels, or impaired fasting glucose or diabetes were analysed and revealed that beta-cell mass was already decreased by 40% in the pre-diabetic state in obese persons and was also decreased in diabetic lean and obese patients. The reduced beta-cell mass was not due to lower neogenesis but rather to an increase in apoptosis. Leahy (2005) has proposed sequences of key pathological features of type 2 diabetes. Both genetic predisposition and environment may play a role in the disease but a third element should appear in the picture which is the acquired defects, in particular the beta-cell dysfunction. The current concept is that both beta-cell dysfunction and insulin resistance occur before the onset of diabetes.

References

Aerts, L. and A. Van Assche (2006). "Animal evidence for the transgenerational development of diabetes mellitus". *Int J Biochem Cell Biol* **38**(5–6): 894–903.

Blondeau, B., J. Lesage, P. Czernichow, J.P. Dupouy and B. Breant (2001). "Glucocorticoids impair fetal beta-cell development in rats". *Am J Physiol Endocrinol Metab* **281**(3): E592–E599.

Boloker J., S.J. Gertz and R.A. Simmons (2002). "Gestational diabetes leads to the development of diabetes in adulthood in the rat". *Diabetes* **51**(5): 1499–1506.

Boujendar, S., E. Arany, D. Hill, C. Remacle and B. Reusens (2003). "Taurine supplementation of a low protein diet fed to rat dams normalized the vascularization of the fetal endocrine pancreas". *J Nutr* **133**(9): 2820–2825.

Butler A.E., J. Janson, S. Bonner-Weir, R. Ritzel, R.A. Rizza and P.C. Butler (2003). "Beta-cell deficit and increased beta-cell apoptosis in human with type 2 diabetes". *Diabetes* **52**(1): 102–110.

Cherif, H., B. Reusens, S. Dahri and C. Remacle (2001). "A protein restricted diet during pregnancy alters in vitro insulin secretion from islets of fetal Wistar rats". *J Nutr* **131**(5): 1555–1559.

Dabelea D., W.C. Knowler and D.J. Pettitt (2000). "Effect of diabetes in pregnancy on offspring: follow-up research in the Pima Indians" *J Mat Fetal Med* **9**(1): 83–88.

Dahri, S., A. Snoeck, B. Reusens, C Remacle and J.J. Hoet (1991). "Islet function in offspring of mothers on low protein diet during gestation". *Diabetes* **40**(suppl 2): 115–120.

Garofano, A., P. Czernichow and B. Bréant (1997). "*In utero* undernutrition impairs rat β-cell development". *Diabetologia* **40**(10): 1231–1234.

Garofano, A., P. Czernichow and B. Bréant (1998). "Beta-cell mass and proliferation following late fetal and early postnatal malnutrition in the rat". *Diabetologia* **41**(9): 1114–1120.

Hales, C.N., D.J. Barker, P.M. Clark, L.J. Cox, C. Fall, C. Osmond and P.D. Winter (1991). "Fetal and infant growth and impaired glucose tolerance at age 64." *BMJ* **303**(6809): 1019–1022.

Innes K.E., T.E. Byers, J.A. Marshall, A. Baron, M. Orleans and R.F. Hamman (2002). "Association of a woman's own birth weight with subsequent risk for gestational diabetes." *JAMA* **287**(19): 2534–2541.

Leahy, J. (2005). "Pathogenesis of type 2 diabetes mellitus". *Arch Med Res* **36**(3): 197–209.

Merezak, S., B. Reusens, M.T. Ahn and C. Remacle (2004). "Effect of maternal low protein diet and taurine on the vulnerability of adult Wistar rat islets to cytokines". *Diabetologia* **47**(4): 669–675.

Molsted-Pedersen, L.L., J. Wagner, L. Klebe and J. Pedersen (1972). "Aspects of carbohydrate metabolism in newborn infants of diabetic mothers. IV. Neonatal changes in plasma free fatty acid concentration." *Acta Endocrinol* **71**: 338–345.

Ozanne, S.E., M.W. Dorling, C.L. Wang and B.T. Nave (2001). "Impaired PI 3-kinase activation in adipocytes from early growth-restricted male rats". *Am J Physiol* **280**(3): E534–E539.

Ozanne, S.E., G.S. Olsen, L.L. Hansen, K.J. Tingey, B.T. Nave, C.L.Wang, K. Hartil, C.J. Petry and L. Mosthaf-Seedorf (2003). "Early growth restriction leads to down regulation of protein kinase C zeta and insulin resistance in skeletal muscle". *J Endocrinol* **177**(2): 235–241.

Ozanne, S.E., C.B. Jensen, K.J. Tingey, H. Stogaard, S. Madbad and A.A. Vaag (2005). "Low birth weight is associated with specific changes in muscle insulin-signalling protein expression". *Diabetologia* **48**(3): 547–552.

Peterside, I.E., M.A. Selak and R.A. Simmons (2003). "Impaired oxidative phosphorylation in hepatic mitochondria in growth-retarded rats". *Am J Physiol Endocrinol Metab* **285**(6): 1258–1266.

Petrik, J., B. Reusens, E. Arany, C. Remacle, C. Coelho, J.J. Hoet and D. Hill (1999). "A low protein diet alters the balance of islet cell replication and apoptosis in the fetal and neonatal rat and is associated with a reduced pancreatic expression of insulin-like growth factor II". *Endocrinology* **140**(10): 4861–4873.

Petry, C.J., M.W. Dorling, D.B. Pawlak, S. Ozanne and C.N. Hales (2001). "Diabetes in old male offspring of rat dams fed a reduced protein diet". *Int J Ex Diabetes Res* **2**(2): 139–143.

Ravelli A.C., J.H. van der Meulen, R.P. Michels, C. Osmond, D.J. Barker, C.N. Hales and O.P. Bleker (1998). "Glucose tolerance in adults after prenatal exposure to famine." *Lancet* **351** (9097): 173–177.

Reusens, B. and C. Remacle (2001). "Intergenerational effects of adverse intrauterine environment on perturbation of glucose metabolism". *Twin Res* **4**(5): 406–411.

Rich-Edwards, J.W., G.A. Colditz, M.J. Stampfer, W.C. Willett, M.W. Gilman, C.H. Hennenkens, F.E. Speizer and J.E. Manson (1999). "Birth-weight and the risk for type 2 diabetes mellitus in adult women." *Ann Int Med* **130**: 278–284.

Simmons, R.A., I. Suponisky-Kroyter and M.A. Selak (2005). "Progressive accumulation of mitochondrial DNA mutations and decline in mitochondrial function lead to beta-cell failure". *J Biol Chem* **280**(31): 28785–28791.

Snoeck, A., C. Remacle, B. Reusens and J.J. Hoet, (1990). "Effect of low protein diet during pregnancy on the fetal rat endocrine pancreas". *Biol Neonate* **57**(2): 107–118.

Sparre, T., B. Reusens, H. Cherif, M.R. Larsen, P. Roepstorff, S.J. Fey, P. Mose Larsen, C. Remacle and J. Nerup (2003). "Intrauterine programming of fetal islet gene expression in rats – effects of maternal protein restriction during gestation revealed by proteome analysis". *Diabetologia* **46**(11): 1497–1511.

Srinivasan M., S.D. Katewa, A. Palaniyappan, J.D. Pandya and M. Patel (2006). "Maternal high-fat diet consumption results in fetal malprogramming predisposing to the onset of metabolic syndrome-like phenotype in adulthood". *Am J Physiol Endocrinol Metab* **291**: E792–E799.

Taylor, P.D., J. McConnell, I.Y. Khan, K. Holemans, K.M. Lawrence, H. Asare-Anane, S.J. Persaud, P. Jones, L. Petrie, M Hanson and L. Poston (2005). "Impaired glucose homeostasis and mitochondrial abnormalities in offspring of rats fed a fat-rich diet in pregnancy". *Am J Physiol Regul Integr Comp Physiol* **288**(1): R134–R139.

Tiedge, M., S. Lortz, J. Drinkgern and S Lenzen (1997). "Relation between antioxidant enzyme gene expression and antioxidative defense status of insulin-producing cells". *Diabetes* **46**(11): 1733–1742.

Van Assche, F.A., F. De Prins, L. Aerts and M. Verjans (1977). "The endocrine pancreas in small for date infants." *Brit J Obst Gynaec* **84**(10): 751–753.

Vickers, M.H., B.H. Breier, W.S. Cutfield, P.L. Hofman and P.D. Gluckman (2000). "Fetal origins of hyperphagia, obesity, and hypertension and postnatal amplification by hypercaloric nutrition". *Am J Physiol Endocrinol Metab* **279**(1): E83–E87.

PGC-1β: A Co-activator That Sets the Tone for Both Basal and Stress-Stimulated Mitochondrial Activity

Christopher J. Lelliott and Antonio Vidal-Puig

Abstract The peroxisomal proliferator-activated receptor-gamma coactivator (PGC) family of transcriptional coactivators are central regulators of a wide-range of metabolic processes, which combine to control whole-body homeostasis. However, the specific function of each PGC in a tissue and pathway-specific context is only now being elucidated. In order to define the specific roles of PGC-1β, we generated a mouse lacking this gene and studied its phenotype using a combination of physiological experiments, guided by a systems biology approach. We found that despite the predicted obese phenotype, PGC1βKO were leaner than wild-type and had elevated energy expenditure in the resting state, probably due to upregulation of a wide-range of oxidative and fuel-handling genes in the brown adipose tissue (BAT), including PGC family member PGC-1α. Nonetheless, we identified that PGC-1β ablation results in a global reduction in oxidative phosphorylation and electron transport chain genes and this translates into mitochondrial dysfunction in selected tissues. PGC1βKO mice also demonstrate blunted responses to physiological stresses such as cold exposure in BAT, adrenergic stimulation in BAT and heart and acute dietary lipid loads in liver. In summary, while lack of PGC-1β is not deleterious, it is essential for the normal expression of mitochondrial metabolic genes and for the optimal ability to handle physiological stresses.

Keywords PGC • mitochondria • brown adipose tissue • knock-out • metabolism

Abbreviations BAT: brown adipose tissue; ETC: electron transport chain; LDL: low density lipoprotein; MVF: mitochondrial volume fraction; NHR: nuclear hormone receptor; PGC: peroxisome proliferator-activated receptor-gamma coactivator;

C.J. Lelliott (✉) and A. Vidal-Puig
Department of Clinical Biochemistry, University of Cambridge, Addenbrooke's Hospital, Hills Road, Cambridge CB2 2QR, UK

C.J. Lelliott
AstraZeneca R&D, SE-431 83 Mölndal, Sweden
christopher.lelliott@astrazeneca.com

B. Koletzko et al. (eds.), *Early Nutrition Programming and Health Outcomes in Later Life: Obesity and Beyond*,

OxPhos: oxidative phosphorylation; VLDL: very-low density lipoprotein; WAT: white adipose tissue; WT: wild type

1 Introduction

Whilst the biochemical pathways underpinning our understanding of metabolism have been known for the last 30 years, it is only within the last decade that we have begun to understand how these pathways are regulated at the transcriptional level. Indeed, in many aspects our knowledge of these processes is far from complete, hence the excitement generated when new factors are identified or when the roles of known proteins are expanded. Whilst much of the focus on the understanding of metabolic gene regulation has been on transcription factors that are able to activate or repress expression of particular genes, more recently transcriptional coactivators and corepressors have been studied in greater and greater depth (Spiegelman and Heinrich 2004; Finck and Kelly 2006).

2 The PGC Family as Metabolic Regulators

Mechanistically, transcriptional coactivators work by acting as a bridge between transcription factors such as nuclear hormone receptors (NHRs) and the rest of the RNA polymerase II transcriptional machinery. They also allow recruitment of factors such as histone acteyltransferases that break down chromatin and allow transcription to occur. The archetypal transcriptional coactivator peroxisomal proliferator-activated receptor-gamma coactivator-1 alpha (PGC-1α), was originally discovered as a physiologically-regulated binding partner for peroxisomal proliferator-activated receptor-gamma PPARγ in brown adipose tissue (BAT) (Puigserver et al. 1998). BAT is a tissue with a high metabolic capacity, since it generates much of the heat required for temperature homeostasis within rodents and functionally needs to be flexible enough to rapidly increase heat production during cold exposure, so-called adaptive thermogenesis. During this process, PGC-1α expression increases in concert with other critical genes required for adaptive thermogenesis such as Uncoupling Protein 1 (UCP1). Overexpression of PGC-1α in many cell types increases mitochondrial biogenesis, mitochondrial gene expression and oxygen consumption (Wu et al. 1999; Lehman et al. 2000; Yoon et al. 2001; St-Pierre et al. 2003).

PGC-1α is now known to be upregulated by other physiological processes such as with fasting in the liver (where it induces gluconeogenesis) (Yoon et al. 2001) and with exercise in skeletal muscle (where is boosts metabolic capacity) (Goto et al. 2000; Baar et al. 2002). Thus PGC-1α provides an excellent example of a transcriptional coactivator with physiological regulation. Since then, we and others have identified a number of other transcriptional coactivators that share homology with PGC-1α. These include PGC1-related coactivator PRC (Andersson and Scarpulla 2001) and PGC-1β/PGC-1 related estrogen receptor coactivator (PERC) (Kressler et al. 2002; Lin et al. 2002; Meirhaeghe et al. 2003). All three family members share a similar basic structure; an N-terminal domain containing nuclear hormone receptor-interacting motifs (LXXLL) and a C-terminal region containing an RNA-binding motif (RMM) and serine-arginine-rich (RS) domains (Lin et al. 2005a). Between these outer domains is a less conserved region which contains different domains and motifs which may be additionally important for the function of each PGC-1 and could provide a method for distinguishing the specificity of each PGC-1, as suggested by the specific interaction of PGC-1β and sterol regulatory element-binding protein-1 (SREBP1) (Lin et al. 2005b). Fitting the role of key regulators of metabolic status, both PGC-1α and PGC-1β are expressed mostly in tissue with high energy consumption, such as skeletal muscle, BAT, heart and brain. PRC on the other hand is ubiquitously expressed.

Much of the early work on PGC-1β focussed on trying to establish its function, especially in relation to PGC-1α. We and others have shown that PGC-1β and PGC-1α share similar properties *in vitro*, as overexpression of either gene results in increased mitochondrial biogenesis and activity (Meirhaeghe et al. 2003; St-Pierre et al. 2003). However, from our studies in rodent models, there were significant differences in the physiological regulation of these PGCs. In conditions where PGC-1α expression is physiologically regulated, PGC-1β expression is relatively unaffected. The only apparent contradiction to this is in acute dietary lipid loads in the liver which PGC-1β is preferentially upregulated (Lin et al. 2005b).

3 Ablation of PGC-1β Results in Metabolic Changes in Multiple Tissues

In an attempt to identify a more specific role of PGC-1β, we generated a mouse lacking a functional *PGC-1β* gene (Lelliott et al. 2006), using a triple LoxP strategy in order to give us the flexibility to generate conditional knock-outs. Since PGC-1β is a relatively promiscuous coactivator, we designed a series of physiological phenotyping protocols in order to identify not only which pathways were specifically affected by the lack of PGC-1β, but also in which tissues and under which conditions. From this data, we then used a systems biology approach to identify altered metabolic pathways, and also to guide a more detailed series of experiments.

3.1 Up-Regulated Genes

Given the expected function of PGC-1β as an important factor in mitochondrial activity, it would be expected that a mouse lacking PGC-1β (PGC1βKO) would be obese. However, our PGC1βKO mouse is leaner than wild-type littermate controls, derived from a reduced amount of white adipose tissue (WAT), rather than lean mass. We also found that minimum oxygen consumption and energy expenditure is raised in the PGC1βKO, in experiments conducted at room temperature (22°C). It is counterintuitive that loss of a coactivator responsible for mitochondrial function should result in increased metabolic rates. Yet gene expression analysis for the BAT from PGC1βKO mice demonstrates that there is a clear global gene expression increase in metabolically-relevant transcription factors (PPARγ1, PPARα), fuel handling proteins (hormone sensitive lipase, Glut4) and uncoupling proteins as well as type 2 deiodinase. PGC-1α expression is also upregulated in BAT from the PGC1βKO mouse, suggesting that there is cross-regulation of the PGC-1s, and that PGC-1α compensates for the absence of PGC-1β in BAT, a finding also seen in WAT.

3.2 Down-Regulated Genes

Despite the upregulation of genes above, genes that are part of the mitochondrial electron transport chain (ETC) and oxidative phosphorylation (OxPhos) were coordinately downregulated. This is a global function of PGC-1β since these are the only downregulated sets of genes common to a range of tissues. Loss of PGC-1β does not necessarily affect the mitochondrial volume fraction (MVF) of a given tissue. Heart and soleus muscle from PGC1βKO mice have a reduced MVF, but this is not the case in BAT, where MVF is equivalent to wild-type levels. Also, BAT is the only one of these three tissues that has a compensatory increase in PGC-1α expression, suggesting that enhanced levels of PGC-1α is sufficient to reverse the reduction in MVF caused by PGC-1β ablation.

4 Altered Response to Physiologic Challenges in PGC1βKO Mice

4.1 In BAT

Given the BAT phenotype above, we examined two further hypotheses. Firstly, being at room temperature (22°C) imparts a thermal stress on mice, so at room temperature BAT is also partially active thermogenically. So since we found that at room temperature, lack of PGC-1β results in a higher minimum energy expenditure, we asked whether PGC-1β ablation results in a changed basal energy expenditure at thermoneutrality (30°C). Secondly, we asked whether PGC-1β is necessary for enhanced BAT adaptive thermogenesis induced by a more severe cold-exposure. Mice were housed at thermoneutrality (30°C) or subjected to stepwise adaptation to 4°C over a period of 7 weeks. Using these adaptive protocols, PGC1βKO mice are cold-tolerant. Measurement of basal energy expenditure at thermoneutrality, showed that in fact PGC-1β ablation results in a reduced basal energy expenditure in both groups of mice. Interestingly, the compensatory increase of PGC-1α in BAT from room-temperature housed PGC1βKO mice was lost in the thermoneutrality-adapted mice, suggesting that the difference in PGC-1α seen at room temperature was induced by the thermal stress at being in a 22°C environment. In cold-adapted mice, BAT PGC-1α levels were similar between wild-type and PGC1βKO. As well as having a reduced basal energy expenditure, both cold-exposed and thermoneutrality-adapted PGC1βKO mice also had an impaired response to norepinephrine, a compound used to drive maximum BAT activity. Thus, PGC-1β is necessary for normal basal energy expenditure and for optimal BAT adaptive thermogenesis.

4.2 In Heart Muscle

Given that our transcriptomic analysis showed that the PGC1βKO mouse has a global defect in genes related to ETC and OxPhos, we examined mitochondrial levels and performance in other tissues. As stated above, in PGC1βKO soleus muscle, MVF is reduced. This is related to reduced ETC/OxPhos gene expression, mitochondrial oxygen expenditure and ATP generation. A similar effect on MVF and ETC/OxPhos gene expression was seen in PGC1βKO hearts. Since the heart requires a large and constant supply of ATP, and must be adaptable to changes in physiological status, the reduction of mitochondrial numbers and in gene expression could be potentially considered deleterious. In order to test this hypothesis, we challenged the mice with dobutamine, a β1,α1-adrenergic selective agonist used to accelerate heart contractions and impose a hemodynamic load onto the muscle. We found that the PGC1βKO mice had normal left ventricular contractility both pre- and post-dobutamine stimulation. However, despite a normal heart rate prior to the intervention, the increase in heart rate after adrenergic stimulation was markedly impaired in the PGC1βKO mice. This suggests that PGC-1β is an important player in the chronotropic mechanism controlling heart rate in response to physiological and chemical stimulus.

4.3 In Liver

It has been previously shown in liver that PGC-1β is important for the handling of acute lipid loads (Lin et al. 2005b; Wolfrum and Stoffel 2006). With short-term saturated fat diets, PGC-1β is upregulated and very-low density lipoprotein (VLDL) output is stimulated to distribute fatty acids into the periphery. Using our PGC1βKO mice we were able to demonstrate that PGC-1β is required for the normal lipid homeostasis in the liver since feeding the PGC1βKO with a short-term saturated fat diet as above caused hepatic lipid accumulation and an increase in liver/body weight ratio due to the lipid infiltration. In addition, PGC1βKO mice have reduced total serum cholesterol, as well as decreased VLDL and low-density lipoprotein (LDL)-cholesterol fractions. This all points towards PGC-1β being a key player for the maintenance of normal cholesterol homeostasis.

5 Lessons from the PGC1βKO Mouse

So what can be learnt from our mouse model about PGC-1β? Perhaps the most important finding was that PGC-1β is a global regulator of the correct levels of mitochondrial gene expression. This is not to say that ablation of PGC-1β is deleterious, at least not in unstressed conditions or in the interventions that we performed with our mice. Indeed, after we published the first report on the PGC1βKO mouse, two other groups have reported that mice with PGC-1β ablated (Sonoda et al. 2007), or a with hypomorphic mutation in PGC-1β (Vianna et al. 2006) do not suffer from overt metabolic failure. Possibly this is due to upregulation of PGC-1α in adipose tissues resulting in a degree of compensation that allows the survival of the mice. This compensation however partially obscures the role of PGC-1β in adipose tissues, whereas we can presume that the true functions of PGC-1β are better illustrated in tissues without PGC-1α compensation, such as heart, liver and skeletal muscle.

In general, the lack of PGC-1β still results in functional tissues, but these tissues work less optimally than normal in basal conditions and with sub-maximal responses to stress stimulation. We hypothesise that PGC-1β and PGC-1α play complementary roles with regards to energy homeostasis. PGC-1β sets the tone for both basal and stress-stimulated mitochondrial activity. On the other hand, upregulation of PGC-1α is necessary during physiological stress to allow the cell to cope with rising energy demands. Future work will allow us to build on this perspective and determine the intricacies of metabolic regulation by transcriptional coactivators.

Acknowledgements The work presented in this paper was supported by the British Heart Foundation, Wellcome Trust Integrative Physiology program and AstraZeneca R&D. The authors would like to thank Gema Medina-Gomez and the other contributors to the studies conducted here.

References

Andersson, U. and R. C. Scarpulla (2001). "Pgc-1-related coactivator, a novel, serum-inducible coactivator of nuclear respiratory factor 1-dependent transcription in mammalian cells." *Mol Cell Biol* **21**(11): 3738–3749.

Baar, K., A. R. Wende, et al. (2002). "Adaptations of skeletal muscle to exercise: rapid increase in the transcriptional coactivator PGC-1." *FASEB J* **16**(14): 1879–1886.

Finck, B. N. and D. P. Kelly (2006). "PGC-1 coactivators: inducible regulators of energy metabolism in health and disease." *J Clin Invest* **116**(3): 615–622.

Goto, M., S. Terada, et al. (2000). "cDNA cloning and mRNA analysis of PGC-1 in epitrochlearis muscle in swimming-exercised rats." *Biochem Biophys Res Commun* **274**(2): 350–354.

Kressler, D., S. N. Schreiber, et al. (2002). "The PGC-1-related protein PERC is a selective coactivator of estrogen receptor alpha." *J Biol Chem* **277**(16): 13918–13925.

Lehman, J. J., P. M. Barger, et al. (2000). "Peroxisome proliferator-activated receptor gamma coactivator-1 promotes cardiac mitochondrial biogenesis." *J Clin Invest* **106**(7): 847–856.

Lelliott, C. J., G. Medina-Gomez, et al. (2006). "Ablation of PGC-1beta results in defective mitochondrial activity, thermogenesis, hepatic function, and cardiac performance." *PLoS Biol* **4**(11): e369.

Lin, J., P. Puigserver, et al. (2002). "Peroxisome proliferator-activated receptor gamma coactivator 1beta (PGC-1beta), a novel PGC-1-related transcription coactivator associated with host cell factor." *J Biol Chem* **277**(3): 1645–1648.

Lin, J., C. Handschin, et al. (2005a). "Metabolic control through the PGC-1 family of transcription coactivators." *Cell Metab* **1**(6): 361–370.

Lin, J., R. Yang, et al. (2005b). "Hyperlipidemic effects of dietary saturated fats mediated through PGC-1beta coactivation of SREBP." *Cell* **120**(2): 261–273.

Meirhaeghe, A., V. Crowley, et al. (2003). "Characterization of the human, mouse and rat PGC1 beta (peroxisome-proliferator-activated receptor-gamma co-activator 1 beta) gene in vitro and in vivo." *Biochem J* **373**(Pt 1): 155–165.

Puigserver, P., Z. Wu, et al. (1998). "A cold-inducible coactivator of nuclear receptors linked to adaptive thermogenesis." *Cell* **92**(6): 829–839.

Sonoda, J., I. R. Mehl, et al. (2007). "PGC-1beta controls mitochondrial metabolism to modulate circadian activity, adaptive thermogenesis, and hepatic steatosis." *Proc Natl Acad Sci USA* **104**(12): 5223–5228.

Spiegelman, B. M. and R. Heinrich (2004). "Biological control through regulated transcriptional coactivators." *Cell* **119**(2): 157–167.

St-Pierre, J., J. Lin, et al. (2003). "Bioenergetic analysis of peroxisome proliferator-activated receptor gamma coactivators 1alpha and 1beta (PGC-1alpha and PGC-1beta) in muscle cells." *J Biol Chem* **278**(29): 26597–26603.

Vianna, C. R., M. Huntgeburth, et al. (2006). "Hypomorphic mutation of PGC-1[beta] causes mitochondrial dysfunction and liver insulin resistance." *Cell Metab* **4**(6): 453.

Wolfrum, C. and M. Stoffel (2006). "Coactivation of Foxa2 through Pgc-1[beta] promotes liver fatty acid oxidation and triglyceride/VLDL secretion." *Cell Metab* **3**(2): 99.

Wu, Z., P. Puigserver, et al. (1999). "Mechanisms controlling mitochondrial biogenesis and respiration through the thermogenic coactivator PGC-1." *Cell* **98**(1): 115–124.

Yoon, J. C., P. Puigserver, et al. (2001). "Control of hepatic gluconeogenesis through the transcriptional coactivator PGC-1." *Nature* **413**(6852): 131–138.

Pharmacological and Gene Modification-Based Models for Studying the Impact of Perinatal Metabolic Disturbances in Adult Life

Francesc Villarroya, Carlos Bocos, Marta Giralt, Maria Pilar Ramos, Emilio Herrera, Julio Sevillano, Margalida Gual, Meritxell Rosell, and Roser Iglesias

Abstract Genetic modification approaches or pharmacological interventions may be useful for understanding the molecular mechanisms by which nutrient derivatives and metabolites exert their effects in the perinatal period and how they may influence long-term metabolism in adults. Examples for such experimental settings in rodents are targeted disruption of the gene for peroxisome proliferator-activated receptor (PPAR)-α, a lipid sensor and master regulator of lipid catabolism, or maternal treatment with agonists of PPARγ, a master regulator of adipogenesis and target of insulin sensitizing drugs in adults. All these interventions show differential effects in the perinatal period compared to adults and indicate that altered activity of master regulators of metabolism results in profound metabolic alterations in the perinatal period that may influence adult metabolism.

Keywords Fetus • fatty acid • insulin sensitivity • neonate • peroxisome proliferator-activated receptor • thiazolidinedione

Abbreviations KO: knock out; PPAR: peroxisome proliferator-activated receptor; TZD: thiazolidinedione; UCP: uncoupling protein

1 Introduction

The primary goal of determining the effects of pre- and post-natal nutrition on offspring development and the potential metabolic disturbances is hampered by the complexities of perinatal nutritional determinants (nutritional components of mater-

F. Villarroya (✉), M. Giralt, M.Gual, M. Rosell, and R. Iglesias
Department of Biochemistry and Molecular Biology and Institut de Biomedicina (IBUB), Universitat de Barcelona, Avda Diagonal 645, 08028-Barcelona, Spain and CIBER Fisiopatologia de la Obesidad y Nutrición, Instituto de Salud Carlos III
fvillarroya@ub.edu

C. Bocos, M.P. Ramos, E. Herrera, and J. Sevillano
Facultad de Farmacia, Universidad San Pablo-CEU, Madrid, Spain

B. Koletzko et al. (eds.), *Early Nutrition Programming and Health Outcomes in Later Life: Obesity and Beyond*,

nal food, placental transfer of metabolites, changes in milk composition, etc.). Thus, together with studies looking at the effects of maternal nutrition on the metabolic outcome of neonates and adults, other complementary approaches have been useful for our advancement in the understanding of the mechanisms and molecular processes driving long-term effects of perinatal nutrition changes. Two experimental approaches in rodent models, not involving nutrition primarily, may be useful: gene manipulation via the generation of transgenic or "knockout" (KO) mice, and pharmacologically-driven action on specific metabolic pathways in the perinatal period.

2 A Gene Manipulation Approach to Perinatal Metabolic Alterations and Their Consequences on Adults: The Example of PPARα-"Knockout" Mice

2.1 The PPAR Family of Nuclear Hormone Receptors

Peroxisome proliferator-activated receptor (PPAR)α is a member of the nuclear hormone receptor superfamily and member of the PPAR family of receptors which includes also PPARγ and PPARβ/δ. PPARα acts as a ligand-dependent transcription factor. It regulates the transcription of genes encoding proteins involved in lipid oxidation and, accordingly, it is expressed in tissues with high levels of fat catabolism such as liver, muscle, heart or brown adipose tissue. The natural ligands of PPARα are fatty acids and some types of leukotrienes. Thus, PPARα is considered a master regulator of lipid catabolism and a sensor of the extent of tissue fatty acid available for oxidation. It constitutes a pivotal molecular link between lipid nutrition components and adaptive regulation of gene expression. Other members of the PPAR family are also regulators of gene expression in relation to lipid metabolism. The function of PPARγ is specifically related to the control of adipogenesis and therefore in lipid accumulation, whereas PPARβ/δ is ubiquitously expressed and it has similar effects to PPARα in promoting fatty acid oxidation (Guri et al. 2006).

2.2 Consequences of Targeted Disruption of PPARα

Multiple metabolic disturbances have been identified in adult mice with targeted disruption of PPARα (PPARα-KO) including impaired adaptation to starvation (hypoglycemica, lowered induction of ketogenesis, etc.), increased fat in liver and adipose tissue under certain dietary challenges but also protection from diet-induced insulin resistance in the context of obesity (Kersten et al. 1999; Leone et al. 1999; Finck et al. 2005). Impaired expression of genes for fatty acid oxidation also takes place in the heart (Murray et al. 2005) but minor alterations occur in skeletal muscle (Muoio et al. 2002). However, it cannot be excluded that disturbances in PPARα-KO adults may result in whole or in part from potential metabolic disturbances due to the lack of PPARα during the fetal or neonatal period and the subsequent effects on metabolism. To clarify this issue, the impact of targeted disruption of PPARα on perinatal metabolism was studied (Yubero et al. 2004; Pedraza et al. 2006). Fetuses from PPARα-KO mice did not show major alterations in circulating metabolites or gene expression in PPARα-expressing tissues when compared with littermates. However, the lack of PPARα had a major impact in the neonatal period. PPARα-KO newborns do not show the increase in ketone levels in blood occurring in wild-type pups whereas they show mild hypoglycemia. An overall impairment in gene expression for enzymes involved in lipid catabolism (hydroxymethylglutharyl-CoA synthase, acyl-CoA oxidase) occur in the liver, whereas no major alterations in gluconeogenic genes (phosphoenolpyruvate carboxykinase, glucose-6-phosphatase) take place (Yubero et al. 2004).

In neonates' hearts, like adults, there are profound changes in gene expression due to the lack of PPARα. They take place shortly after the initiation of suckling but do not occur just at birth. For instance, PPARα-KO neonates show impaired expression of genes which are induced in wild-type pups as a consequence of initiation of milk intake (such as uncoupling proteins [UCP] 2 and 3, pyruvate-dehydrogenase kinase-4, or carnitine palmitoyl-transferase II) (Pedraza et al. 2006). Skeletal muscle appears to be much less sensitive to the lack of PPARα, and only UCP3 and UCP2 gene expression was impaired in PPARα-KO neonates. However, this was different from adults, in which skeletal muscle gene expression appears to be unaltered for both genes. The most likely explanation for these differences in skeletal muscle gene expression between adults and neonates is a redundant compensatory effect of PPARβ/δ, which may share target genes with PPARα. It is not clear why this compensation occurs only in skeletal muscle from adults and not from neonates or why this does not happen in the heart. Developmental regulation of gene expression for PPARα and PPARβ/δ in these tissues can hardly be an explanation. In skeletal muscle, PPARα gene expression is low in fetuses but it is highly induced just before birth. Neonates show high levels of PPARα gene expression and a progressive decline thereafter. Thus, PPARα gene expression is much lower in neonates than in adults (Brun et al. 1999). In contrast, PPARβ/δ gene expression in muscle is unchanged when neonates and adults are compared. Thus, in some sense, PPARα expression is more prevalent compared to PPARβ/δ in the neonate than in the adult, and this may explain the particular sensitivity of neonatal skeletal muscle to the lack of PPARα. However, PPARα gene expression in heart is similar in neonates and adults whereas PPARβ/δ is more expressed in adults than in neonates (Pedraza et al. 2006). There is no dramatic difference in the extent of PPARβ/δ expression in skeletal muscle and heart that could explain why compensatory mechanisms may be more efficient in muscle than in heart.

Another tissue showing relevant alterations in gene expression during the neonatal period is brown fat. The naturally-occurring induction of genes involved in fatty acid oxidation after birth is reduced in PPARα-KO mice, and also UCP1 gene, the pivotal gene for induction of thermogenesis, is down-regulated in PPARα-KO neonates

(M. Rosell and R. Iglesias, 2007). This is consistent with the identification of UCP1 as a target gene of PPARα-dependent transcriptional control (Barbera et al. 2001).

2.3 *The Effect of Milk Intake on Neonatal Metabolism*

The profound disturbances in tissues and systemic metabolism in PPARα-KO neonates can be explained by the sudden requirement of fatty acid catabolism after birth. During pregnancy, glucose coming from placental transfer is the main source of metabolic energy for fetuses. However, after birth, due to the fact that milk in rodents contains large amounts of fat, neonates experience the sudden requirement to activate genes encoding the enzymatic machinery of fatty acid catabolism Thus, the adaptations in fuel usage taking place in adults as a consequence of starvation occur in neonates as a consequence of milk intake. Thus, in neonates with targeted disruption of PPARα, there is an impaired usage of milk fatty acids by liver, as evidenced by the impaired induction of ketogenesis. Peripheral usage of fatty acids is also impaired, as indicated by the reduction in gene expression for fatty acid catabolism genes in heart, muscle and brown adipose tissue (Fig. 1). This observation confirms the importance of PPARα in the control of neonatal thermogenesis. Fatty acid oxidation provides the fuel for thermogenesis to support uncoupled oxidation in brown fat mitochondria and the subsequent heat production. Although the lack of PPARα does not lead to a deep reduction in thermogenesis that challenges neonatal survival, it is expected that PPARα-KO neonates experience, together

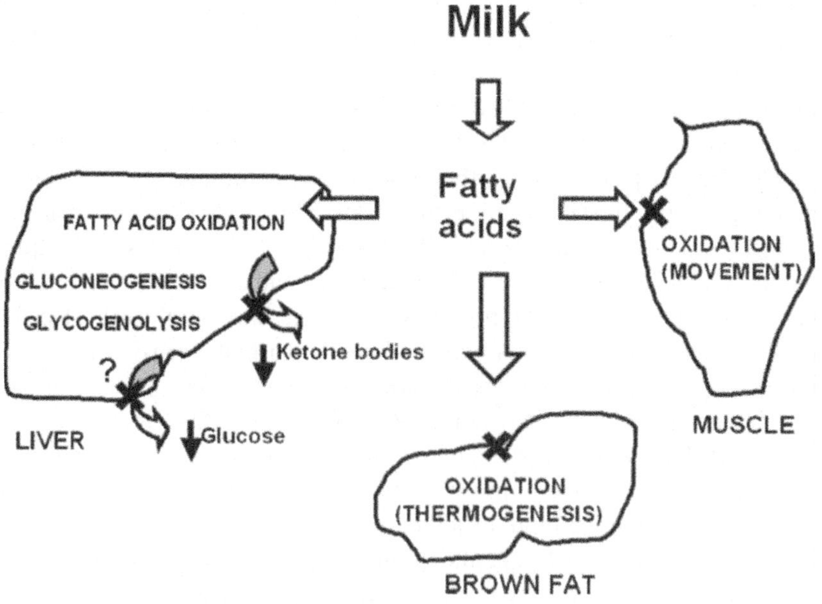

Fig. 1 Metabolic fate of milk derived fatty acids during suckling and disruption caused by the lack of PPARα. The X marks indicate metabolic consequences of impaired fatty acid utilization due to the lack of PPARα in suckling neonates

with an overall impairment of metabolic fuel usage reminiscent of undernutrition, a transient impairment in the control of body temperature.

2.4 *Implications for Future Studies*

These profound alterations in PPARα-KO neonates also have important overall implications for experimental studies using targeted disruption of genes to analyze their function in metabolism. It is essential that adult mice with targeted disruption of a given gene are always studied in comparison with wild-type controls that do not experience any gene disruption-mediated alteration in nutrition during pregnancy or lactation. For instance, using the PPARα-KO mice as example, the comparison of adult PPARα-KO mice with wild-type controls, each one kept on separate mice strains and therefore experiencing differential exposure to maternal metabolic alterations during pregnancy or lactation, is not correct. Despite the almost complete absence of direct studies, it may be expected that the lack of PPARα, a master gene of lipid metabolism, may affect maternal lipid metabolism, milk composition and even mammary gland development (Yang et al. 2006). Changes in the metabolic status of PPARα-KO adults may therefore be the result not of the intrinsic effects of the lack of PPARα on adult metabolic regulation but of the long-term effects of altered perinatal metabolism.

Thus, it is essential that maternal behaviour and nutritional delivery to fetuses and pups are the same if strict analysis of the effects of disruption of a given gene in adults is to be undertaken. A potential approach would be to compare wild-type and PPARα-KO littermates raised by mating male and female PPARα-KO heterozygotes. In such case, although maternal pregnancy and lactation will be performed by an heterozygote female, it would be at least common to wild-type and PPARα-KO littermates. A further control of these aspects, although of a higher experimental complexity, will be the use of wild-type foster mothers to lactate litters composed of wild-type and PPARα-KO pups to ensure a common normal lactation. However, ultimate differential nutrition during lactation caused by a potential effect of the lack of PPARα on suckling behaviour would not be controlled by these experimental settings.

3 A Pharmacological Approach to the Effects of Perinatal Metabolic Alterations and Their Consequences in Adults: The Effects of a PPARγ Agonist During Pregnancy on Neonatal and Adult Rats

Another potential way of investigating the effects of metabolic disturbances during the perinatal period on adults using non-nutritional approaches is to modulate targets of nutritional regulation by means of specific drugs. An example of such approach would be the analysis of the action of thiazolidinediones (TZDs) during pregnancy on neonatal and adult life. TZDs are used as anti-diabetic drugs in adults because they ameliorate insulin resistance. TZDs act as activators of PPARγ, the member of the PPAR family of transcription factors expressed preferentially in adipose tissues and involved in promoting adipocyte differentiation.

Pregnant rats were treated for 4 days with an oral dose of 50 mg of the TZD englitazone/kg of body mass daily from day 16 of gestation. Neonates from englitazone-treated pregnant rats showed insulin-resistance, as evidenced by reduced glucose/insulin ratio, high free fatty acid levels, enhanced ketonaemia and low plasma IGF-I levels. In liver, lipoprotein lipase activity and Akt phosphorylation were increased (Sevillano et al. 2005). A profound alteration occurred in brown adipose tissue from neonates: there was a massive accumulation of triacylglycerols in the tissue together with an overall repression of specific marker genes of brown versus white adipose tissue phenotype such as UCP1, PPARγ-coactivator-1α or cytochrome oxidase subunit IV (M. Gual, J. Sevillano, and C. Bocos, 2007) Thus, the response of neonates to maternal antidiabetic drug treatment is the opposite of what would be expected and this may have consequences on the adult. In fact, preliminary data studying neonates who experienced the maternal treatment with the TZD during pregnancy, indicate permanent systemic alterations as well as disturbances in adipose tissue development in the adult life. There are several hypothesis that could be considered to explain the profound effects of TZD treatment during pregnancy on neonatal metabolism. First, it should be considered that some extent of insulin resistance is part of the maternal metabolic adaptations to pregnancy, and TZDs would impair the physiological insulin resistance associated with gestation. It is considered that such insulin resistance in pregnancy favours the channelling of glucose to the fetuses and the alternative usage of other fuels by maternal tissues. However, there are no clear signs of lack of glucose availability in fetuses from treated mothers and, in fact, lipid accumulation in brown adipose tissue is likely to result from enhanced lipogenesis from glucose in the late fetal period. Transient reductions in glucose availability after each TZD administration may increase fetal insulin and therefore activate the lipogenic pathway. Another possibility is a direct effect of englitazone on fetal development. Although not extensively studied, TZDs are considered to be capable of crossing the placenta (O'Moore-Sullivan and Prins 2002). and therefore they may act directly on target genes through PPARγ activation in fetal tissues. Fetuses do not possess white fat and brown fat is probably the main site of PPARγ gene expression in fetuses. It may be suggested that the lack of the main site of action of PPARγ activation in the adult, white fat, may be responsible for the lack of anti-diabetic effect of TZDs in the perinatal period. However, it is clear that brown fat responds to the treatment in a way reminiscent of transdifferentiation into a "white fat-like" phenotype. How this may influence overall insulin sensitivity and cause insulin resistance in neonates deserves further study. In any case, the response of brown adipose tissue in developing fetuses to englitazone cannot be explained solely as a direct effect because *in vitro* treatment of brown pre-adipocytes with englitazone does not impair brown fat-specific gene expression but rather the opposite, and enhances it (M. Rosell & M. Gual, 2007).

4 Conclusions

In summary, it is possible, either by genetic modification or pharmacological intervention, to act during the perinatal period on master regulators of metabolism that, like PPARs, behave as intracellular sensors of nutritional signals. Such experimental approaches may help to delineate the molecular events that may be disturbed as a consequence of altered perinatal nutrition that would cause long-standing consequences in adult metabolism.

Acknowledgments Supported by grants from Ministerio de Educación y Ciencia (SAF2005-01722), Fondo de Investigaciones Sanitarias, Ministerio de Sanidad y Consumo (PI052336 and PI060352) and Universidad San Pablo-CEU (PC10/06). Spain.

References

Barbera MJ, Schluter A, Pedraza N, Iglesias R, Villarroya F, Giralt M (2001). Peroxisome proliferator-activated receptor alpha activates transcription of the brown fat uncoupling protein-1 gene. A link between regulation of the thermogenic and lipid oxidation pathways in the brown fat cell. *J Biol Chem* **276**(2): 1486–1493.

Brun S, Carmona MC, Mampel T, Vinas O, Giralt M, Iglesias R, Villarroya F (1999). Activators of peroxisome proliferator-activated receptor-alpha induce the expression of the uncoupling protein-3 gene in skeletal muscle: a potential mechanism for the lipid intake-dependent activation of uncoupling protein-3 gene expression at birth. *Diabetes* **48**(6): 1217–1222.

Finck BN, Bernal-Mizrachi C, Han DH, Coleman T, Sambandam N, LaRiviere LL, Holloszy JO, Semenkovich CF, Kelly DP (2005). A potential link between muscle peroxisome proliferator-activated receptor-alpha signaling and obesity-related diabetes. *Cell Metab* **1**(2): 133–144.

Guri AJ, Hontecillas R, Bassaganya-Riera J (2006). Peroxisome proliferator-activated receptors: bridging metabolic syndrome with molecular nutrition. *Clin Nutr* **25**(6): 871–885.

Kersten S, Seydoux J, Peters JM, Gonzalez FJ, Desvergne B, Wahli W (1999). Peroxisome proliferator-activated receptor alpha mediates the adaptive response to fasting. *J Clin Invest* **103**(11): 1489–1498.

Leone TC, Weinheimer CJ, Kelly DP (1999). A critical role for the peroxisome proliferator-activated receptor alpha (PPARalpha) in the cellular fasting response: the PPARalpha-null mouse as a model of fatty acid oxidation disorders. *Proc Natl Acad Sci USA* **96**(13): 7473–7478.

Muoio DM, MacLean PS, Lang DB, Li S, Houmard JA, Way JM, Winegar DA, Corton JC, Dohm GL, Kraus WE (2002). Fatty acid homeostasis and induction of lipid regulatory genes in skeletal muscles of peroxisome proliferator-activated receptor (PPAR) alpha knock-out mice. Evidence for compensatory regulation by PPAR delta. *J Biol Chem* **277**(29): 26089–26097.

Murray AJ, Panagia M, Hauton D, Gibbons GF, Clarke K (2005). Plasma free fatty acids and peroxisome proliferator-activated receptor alpha in the control of myocardial uncoupling protein levels. *Diabetes* **54**(12): 3496–3502.

O'Moore-Sullivan TM, Prins JB (2002). Thiazolidinediones and type 2 diabetes: new drugs for an old disease. *Med J Aust* **176**(8): 381–386.

Pedraza N, Rosell M, Villarroya J, Iglesias R, Gonzalez FJ, Solanes G, Villarroya F (2006). Developmental and tissue-specific involvement of peroxisome proliferator-activated receptor-alpha in the control of mouse uncoupling protein-3 gene expression. *Endocrinology* **147**(10): 4695–4704.

Sevillano J, Lopez-Perez IC, Herrera E, Del Pilar Ramos M, Bocos C (2005). Englitazone administration to late pregnant rats produces delayed body growth and insulin resistance in their fetuses and neonates. *Biochem J* **389**(Pt 3): 913–918.

Yang Q, Kurotani R, Yamada A, Kimura S, Gonzalez FJ (2006). Peroxisome proliferator-activated receptor alpha activation during pregnancy severely impairs mammary lobuloalveolar development in mice. *Endocrinology* **147**(10): 4772–4780.

Yubero P, Hondares E, Carmona MC, Rossell M, Gonzalez FJ, Iglesias R, Giralt M, Villarroya F (2004). The developmental regulation of peroxisome proliferator-activated receptor-gamma coactivator-1alpha expression in the liver is partially dissociated from the control of gluconeogenesis and lipid catabolism. *Endocrinology* **145**(9): 4268–4277.

Adipose Tissue–Muscle Interactions and the Metabolic Effects of n-3 LCPUFA – *Implications for Programming Effects of Early Diet*

Petra Janovska and Jan Kopecky

Abstract Studies in adult animals as well as in humans have demonstrated beneficial effects of increased intake of n-3 long-chain polyunsaturated fatty acids (n-3 LCPUFA) on lipid metabolism, obesity, and insulin sensitivity. The lipid composition of breast milk, and in particular, the role of n-3 LCPUFA in imprinting of metabolism and its hormonal control need clarification as far as the long-term beneficial effects of breastfeeding on health are concerned. In this respect, animal studies have brought inconclusive results. However, the involvement of adipose tissue–muscle interactions in the short term effects of n-3 LCPUFA during perinatal development, as well as the lasting effects of n-3 LCPUFA intake, are likely to occur and should be further investigated.

Keywords Adipose tissue • muscle • imprinting • n-3 polyunsaturated fatty acids • obesity • insulin sensitivity

Abbreviations AA: arachidonic acid; ALA: alpha-linolenic acid; AMPK: adenosine monophosphate-activated protein kinase; DHA: docosahexaenoic acid; EPA: eicosapentaenoic acid; HNF-4: hepatic nuclear factor-4; LA: linoleic acid; LCPUFA: long-chain (≥20 carbon atoms) polyunsaturated fatty acids; LXR: liver-X factor α; PPAR: peroxisome proliferator-activated receptors; SCD1: stearoyl-CoA desaturase 1; SREBP-1: sterol regulatory element binding protein-1

1 Introduction – LCPUFAs

The long-term beneficial effects of breastfeeding on health are likely to be related, at least in part, to the lipid composition of breast milk. In particular, the long-chain (≥20 carbon atoms) polyunsaturated fatty acids (LCPUFA) of both n-3 and n-6 series,

P. Janovska and J. Kopecky (✉)
Department of Adipose Tissue Biology, the Institute of Physiology of the Academy of Sciences of the Czech Republic, v.v.i., Videnska 1083, 142 20 Prague, Czech Republic
kopecky@biomed.cas.cz

B. Koletzko et al. (eds.), *Early Nutrition Programming and Health Outcomes in Later Life: Obesity and Beyond*,

i.e. docosahexaenoic acid (DHA; 22:6n-3) and arachidonic acid (AA; 20:4n-3), are crucial components of the milk, because: (i) their role in development has been documented; (ii) neither DHA and AA, nor their precursors, alpha-linolenic acid (ALA; 18:3n-3) and linoleic acid (LA; 18:2n-6), respectively, can be synthesized in human body and must come from food; and (iii) rate of conversion of ALA and LA into LCPUFA is relatively low in the newborn, therefore LCPUFA rather than their precursors represent essential fatty acids during the human perinatal development (Hadders-Algra 2005; Uauy et al. 2003). In spite of these facts, optimization of LCPUFA intake by pregnant mothers, as well as supplementation of formula for neonates by LCPUFA represents an important challenge in neonatology, especially with regard to possible differences in requirements for LCPUFA intake between mature and premature neonates. A better understanding of the mechanisms of the effects of LCPUFA may improve the nutritional supplementation strategies for both the mother and the neonate.

The effects of LCPUFA in development are considered to be very complex. Thus, intake of LCPUFA during perinatal period may have lasting beneficial effects on neurodevelopmental outcome, consistent with the high content of DHA in brain and retina (Hadders-Algra 2005). It has been hypothesized that LCPUFA are also involved in the anti-obesity (Arenz et al. 2004) and anti-diabetic effects (Knip and Akerblom 2005) of breastfeeding. In this respect, the role of eicosapentaenoic acid (EPA; 20:5n-3) should also be considered. EPA, together with DHA, represent the main biologically active fatty acids in sea food and fish oil, it is more abundant than DHA in most sea fish products and n-3 (omega 3) PUFA supplements, and it is essential for the beneficial effects of fish oil in adults. Thus, it has been demonstrated that fish oil and EPA/DHA concentrates prevented the development of obesity (Ruzickova et al. 2004; Flachs et al. 2005) and insulin resistance (Storlien et al. 1987) in rodents fed a high-fat diet. In adult humans, EPA/DHA act as hypolipidemics, reduce cardiac events, and decrease progression of atherosclerosis (reviewed in Ruxton et al. [2004]). Several studies in obese humans demonstrated reduction of adiposity after n-3 LCPUFA supplementation (Couet et al. 1997; Kunesova et al. 2006). However, numerous studies on diabetic patients have demonstrated that n-3 LCPUFA are not able to reverse already established insulin resistance. The reason for the lack of efficiency of n-3 LCPUFA in this respect is not known. The role of n-3 LCPUFA in the prevention of diabetes, and possibly also in the imprinting of insulin sensitivity and glucose homeostasis, needs further investigation.

The metabolic effects of n-3 LC-PUFA are largely mediated by transcription factors, peroxisome proliferator-activated receptors (PPARs), with PPAR-α and PPAR-δ (-β) representing the main target for n-3 LCPUFA; as well as by liver-X factor α (LXR), hepatic nuclear factor-4 (HNF-4), and sterol regulatory element binding protein-1 (SREBP-1); (Madsen et al. 2005). Besides acting directly, most of the effects of n-3 LCPUFA are mediated indirectly through their active metabolites, the eicosanoids (Madsen et al. 2005), and other lipid molecules (Serhan 2005). Mainly through the action of these metabolites, n-3 LCPUFA may reduce inflammation, including the low grade inflammatory response of adipose tissue associated with obesity (J.K. Kuda 2008). The hypolipidemic and anti-obesity effects of n-3 LCPUFA probably depend on the suppression of lipogenesis and the increase in fatty acid oxidation in the liver (Madsen et al. 2005) and the modulation of glucose homeostasis including suppression of liver gluconeogenesis. However, the anti-diabetic effect also reflects modulation of adipose tissue and muscle metabolism and insulin sensitivity of these tissues (see below).

2 Adipose Tissue and n-3 LCPUFA

White adipose tissue represents an important player involved in the effect of PUFA because:

1. It stores fatty acids including PUFA in their most concentrated form, i.e. incorporated into molecules of triglycerides. Thus, the adipose tissue of the mother serves as a buffer for LCPUFA and prevents large fluctuations of LCPUFA concentrations in milk (Fidler et al. 2000).
2. Since mitochondrial biogenesis and β-oxidation of fatty acids in white fat of adult rodents are enhanced specifically by n-3 LCPUFA (Flachs et al. 2005; Madsen et al. 2005), n-3 LCPUFA reduce toxic accumulation of fatty acids in muscle and other tissues (lipotoxicity) and prevent development of insulin resistance induced by increased fat intake.
3. Intake of n-3 LCPUFA induces release of insulin-sensitizing hormone adiponectin from white fat cells of adult rodents *via* PPAR-γ that interacts with adiponectin gene promoter (Flachs et al. 2006); this may be an important mechanism by which n-3 LCPUFA prevent the high-fat diet induced impairment of glucose homeostasis in rodent species. In human breast milk, adiponectin levels are related to nutritional variables of mothers (Bronsky et al. 2006) and, therefore, may be induced by n-3 LCPUFA targetting the adipose tissue of the mother. Consequently, adiponectin from milk may affect the gastrointestinal tract of the newborn and may be involved in the protective effects of breastfeeding. The main source of adiponectin for the fetus during its intrauterine development is probably the placenta (Chen et al. 2006).

Our results from experiments in adult mice fed a high-fat diet (based on corn oil) have demonstrated that n-3 LCPUFA intake prevented the proliferation of adipose tissue cells (Ruzickova et al. 2004). This anti-proliferative effect of n-3 LCPUFA may be involved in the reduced adiposity of pups born to rat or mouse dams that were fed diets supplemented by n-3 LCPUFA (Korotkova et al. 2002) or ALA (Massiera et al. 2003) during gestation and suckling. The decrease in adiposity may explain reduced leptin levels in the rat offspring (Korotkova et al. 2002).

During the perinatal period, dynamic recruitment of both brown and white fat occurs, with important differences among species. Human newborns, similarly to guinea pigs and lambs, are born with substantial amounts of both tissues, with brown and white fat developed during the last trimester of gestation (Merklin 1974; Houstek et al. 1993). On the other hand, in commonly used experimental laboratory rodents like mice and rats, brown fat starts to develop just before birth (Houstek et al. 1988) and white adipose tissue develops mainly postnatally (Herrera and Amusquivar 2000), with subcutaneous fat development preceding that of white fat in the abdomen. Therefore, mice and rats do not represent an ideal model for studies on humans adipose tissue perinatal development and the systemic role of the tissue and other animal models may be used instead (see above and Mace et al. 2006).

It has been proposed that the type of fat consumed affects adipose tissue development and that a relatively high intake of n-6 as compared with n-3 PUFA during pregnancy, the suckling period, and early infancy could lead to childhood obesity (Massiera et al. 2003). This may be of special importance for modern human society facing an increase of n-6/n-3 PUFA ratio in the diet (Korotkova et al. 2002; Massiera et al. 2003). However, the presumptions about the role of n-6/n-3 PUFA ratio in determining adipose tissue development are derived only from experiments in mice, they have not been supported by experiments in other species (Mace et al. 2006), and further studies are required.

3 Muscle and n-3 LCPUFA

Muscle is the most important site of whole body lipid and glucose oxidation. In contrast to the direct effects of n-3 LCPUFA on gene expression and metabolism in adipose tissue and liver, and also on the secretion of adiponectin, the effects of these compounds in muscles are mostly indirect. The preventive effects of EPA and DHA on the development of insulin resistance in muscles of rodents fed high-fat diet correlates well with the decrease of muscle triglyceride content (Storlien et al. 1991). This most probably results from the hypolipidemic effect of EPA and DHA, reflecting the decrease in lipogenesis and increase in lipid oxidation in both liver and adipose tissue (see above). Both adiponectin (Yamauchi et al. 2002) and leptin (Minokoshi et al. 2002) released from adipose tissue augment the oxidation of fatty acids in myocytes and the influx of glucose into these cells *via* an intracellular regulatory pathway, the adenosine monophosphate-activated protein kinase (AMPK). The AMPK pathway evolved to secure energy status of cells and to activate a switch from a glycolytic to an oxidative pattern of energy conversion. Therefore, the role of the AMPK pathway in the control of the changing pattern of energy metabolism during the perinatal development should be studied. That the AMPK regulatory pathway may be involved in the impaired postnatal activation of mitochondrial metabolism by nutritional lipids in muscles of very preterm newborns was demonstrated by our group recently (Brauner et al. 2006). Our experiments in mice suggested the involvement of the leptin – AMPK axes in a strain-specific induction of oxygen consumption in an oxidative type of skeletal muscle by weaning onto a high-fat diet, which was detected in obesity-resistant A/J mice and not in obesity-prone C57BL/6 mice. These studies (J.K. Kus 2008) also support an emerging role of stearoyl-CoA desaturase 1 (SCD1) in the control of lipid oxidation in the muscle, its action as a downstream component of the leptin signaling pathway, and the use of SCD1 expression as a sensitive marker of the activity of tissue lipid metabolism (Dobrzyn and Dobrzyn 2006).

n-3 LCPUFA could also affect muscle directly, independently of their action upon adipose tissue. The direct effects depend on accumulation of n-3 LCPUFA in phospholipids of cell membranes, modulation of the metabolism of eicosanoids, and on modulation of gene expression (*via* PPARs and other transcriptional mechanisms in muscle cells) by n-3 LCPUFA. DHA, especially, is known to accumulate in the cell membranes, and hence change their physical properties. These changes may also affect insulin signaling (Lombardo and Chicco 2006). A protective effect of n-3 LCPUFA against insulin resistance induced by high-fat diets in rat muscle correlated with the DHA content in muscle phospholipids (Storlien et al. 1991). Conversion of EPA and DHA into eicosanoids requires the release of n-3 LC-PUFA from membrane phospholipids.

4 Long-Lasting Effects of n-3 LCPUFA on Energy and Glucose Homeostasis

In spite of a general opinion that dietary intake of n-3 LCPUFA during gestation, lactation, and weaning may have long-lasting (imprinting) effects on energy metabolism, propensity to obesity and control of glucose homeostasis, experimental evidence in this respect is weak and controversial (Waterland and Rached 2006). With respect to the imprinting, n-3 LCPUFA have been reported to exert positive (Massiera et al. 2003; Chapman et al. 2000; Siemelink et al. 2002), as well as no (Mace et al. 2006; Herrera et al. 2005) effects. Studies on the role of n-3 LCPUFA in imprinting are perhaps hampered by a lack of appropriate experimental models. Thus, while the metabolic effects of n-3 LCPUFA are studied successfully in adult laboratory rodents like rats and mice (see above), these laboratory species are not ideally suited for the studies on the imprinting by n-3 LCPUFA. This type of imprinting may depend in large on the adipose tissue–muscle interactions, while perinatal development of adipose tissue in these species is much delayed compared with the human situation (see above). Moreover, it has been observed that intake of n-3 LCPUFA in rats and mice was associated with lower food intake during pregnancy (Siemelink et al. 2002), reduced milk yield of dams (Herrera et al. 2005), as well as with lower body weight of neonates during the whole suckling period (Korotkova et al. 2002; Siemelink et al. 2002; Herrera et al. 2005), and with smaller litter size at birth (Siemelink et al. 2002; P. Janovska and J. Kopecky 2008). A recent carefully performed study (Herrera et al. 2005) suggested that reduced pancreatic glucose responsiveness to insulin release in adult rat offsprings, that were suckled by dams fed a fish oil diet, resulted from decreased food intake rather than the change of milk composition during suckling. In fact, in analogy with the effect of a synthetic PPAR-γ agonists administrated during the late intrauterine development of the rat (Sevillano et al. 2005), also intake of n-3 LCPUFA during this period may cause insulin resistance of the offspring, due to preferential hepatic effects, in the absence of the adipose tissue target (Sevillano et al. 2005). It may be speculated that, due to the relatively late development of adipose tissue during ontogeny of rats and mice, these species are better suited to serve as models for studying the role of n-3 LCPUFA in imprinting occurring during postweaning period rather than during gestation and lactation.

Perhaps, the best example at the moment of the involvement of the adipose tissue–muscle interactions in imprinting is the prevention of diet-induced obesity and impaired glucose tolerance in rats following administration of leptin to their mothers (Stocker et al. 2007), also in agreement with the effect of milk-borne maternal leptin providing protection against obesity to human infants (Miralles et al. 2006). That n-3 LCPUFA intake during gestation and lactation in rats lowered rather than increased serum leptin of the pups (Korotkova et al. 2002) should warrant further investigations (see above). Important interactions between the effects of n-3 LCPUFA and impaired nutrition during intrauterine development on the imprinting of the propensity to obesity (Yura et al. 2005) may be found. Recent studies suggested that epigenetic modulation of the transcriptional machinery in both adipose tissue and liver may be involved, with PPAR-α serving as a lipid sensor and representing the key regulatory element (Waterland and Rached 2006; Bispham et al. 2005; Lillycrop et al. 2005) and references therein.

5 Conclusions

Taking into the consideration numerous beneficial effects of n-3 LCPUFA on metabolism and glucose homeostasis, well documented in adult animals and humans and including the adipose tissue–muscle interactions, similar short-term effects should be expected to occur also during perinatal development. In order to verify existence of these effects, and to assess their possible long-lasting consequences, improvements of the currently used experimental animal models are necessary. Using mild dosage of n-3 LCPUFA in the diet, by selecting the appropriate time for n-3 LCPUFA administration during the perinatal development, and by using appropriate animal species, it may be possible to separate the effects of n-3 LCPUFA on food intake and milk production from their effects on gene expression, and metabolism in tissues, and eventually whole body phenotypes. Since molecular basis of the epigenetic gene regulation remains uncertain (Waterland and Rached 2006), and the effects on complex phenotypes like propensity to obesity or sensitivity to insulin may be masked by array of compensatory mechanisms, analysis of simple markers of the n-3 LCPUFA action in tissues should be performed. These markers may include composition of tissues, as well as expression of selected genes, like SCD1 and PPAR-α.

Acknowledgements We thank Pavel Flachs for critical reading of the manuscript. Unpublished studies mentioned in the text were supported in part by the European Commission (FOOD-CT-2005-007036).

References

Arenz, S., Ruckerl, R., Koletzko, B., and Von Kries, R. (2004). "Breast-feeding and childhood obesity – a systematic review." *Int J Obes Relat Metab Disord* **28**(10), 1247–1256.

Bispham, J., Gardner, D. S., Gnanalingham, M. G., Stephenson, T., Symonds, M. E., and Budge, H. (2005). "Maternal nutritional programming of fetal adipose tissue development: differential effects on messenger ribonucleic acid abundance for uncoupling proteins and peroxisome proliferator-activated and prolactin receptors." *Endocrinology* **146**(9), 3943–3949.

Brauner, P., Kopecky, P., Flachs, P., Kuda, O., Vorlicek, J., Planickova, L., Vitkova, I., Andreelli, F., Foretz, M., Viollet, B., and Kopecky, J. (2006). "Expression of uncoupling protein 3 and GLUT4 gene in skeletal muscle of preterm newborns: possible control by AMP-activated protein kinase." *Pediatr Res* **60**(5), 569–575.

Bronsky, J., Karpisek, M., Bronska, E., Pechova, M., Jancikova, B., Kotolova, H., Stejskal, D., Prusa, R., and Nevoral, J. (2006). "Adiponectin, adipocyte fatty acid binding protein, and epidermal fatty acid binding protein: proteins newly identified in human breast milk." *Clin Chem* **52**(9), 1763–1770.

Chapman, C., Morgan, L. M., and Murphy, M. C. (2000). "Maternal and early dietary fatty acid intake: changes in lipid metabolism and liver enzymes in adult rats." *J Nutr* **130**(2), 146–151.

Chen, J., Tan, B., Karteris, E., Zervou, S., Digby, J., Hillhouse, E. W., Vatish, M., and Randeva, H. S. (2006). "Secretion of adiponectin by human placenta: differential modulation of adiponectin and its receptors by cytokines." *Diabetologia* **49**(6), 1292–1302.

Couet, C., Delarue, J., Ritz, P., Antoine, J.-M., and Lamisse, F. (1997). "Effect of dietary fish oil on body fat mass and basal fat oxidation in healthy adults." *Int J Obes Relat Metab Disord* **21**(8), 637–643.

Dobrzyn, A. and Dobrzyn, P. (2006). "Stearoyl-CoA desaturase – a new player in skeletal muscle metabolism regulation." *J Physiol Pharmacol* **57**(Suppl 10), 31–42.

Fidler, N., Sauerwald, T., Pohl, A., Demmelmair, H., and Koletzko, B. (2000). "Docosahexaenoic acid transfer into human milk after dietary supplementation: a randomized clinical trial." *J Lipid Res* **41**(9), 1376–1383.

Flachs, P., Horakova, O., Brauner, P., Rossmeisl, M., Pecina, P., Franssen-van Hal, N. L., Ruzickova, J., Sponarova, J., Drahota, Z., Vlcek, C., Keijer, J., Houstek, J., and Kopecky, J. (2005). "Polyunsaturated fatty acids of marine origin upregulate mitochondrial biogenesis and induce beta-oxidation in white fat." *Diabetologia* **48**(11), 2365–2375.

Flachs, P., Mohamed-Ali, V., Horakova, O., Rossmeisl, M., Hosseinzadeh-Attar, M. J., Hensler, M., Ruzickova, J., and Kopecky, J. (2006). "Polyunsaturated fatty acids of marine origin induce adiponectin in mice fed high-fat diet." *Diabetologia* **49**(2), 394–397.

Hadders-Algra, M. (2005). "The role of long-chain polyunsaturated fatty acids (LCPUFA) in growth and development." *Adv Exp Med Biol* **569**, 80–94.

Herrera, E. and Amusquivar, E. (2000). "Lipid metabolism in the fetus and the newborn." *Diabetes Metab Res Rev* **16**(3), 202–210.

Herrera, E., Lopez-Soldado, I., Limones, M., Amusquivar, E., and Ramos, M. P. (2005). "Experimental models for studying perinatal lipid metabolism. Long-term effects of perinatal undernutrition." *Adv Exp Med Biol* **569**, 95–108.

Houstek, J., Vizek, K., Pavelka, S., Kopecky, J., Krejcova, E., Hermanska, E., and Cermakova, S. (1993). "Type II iodothyronine 5′-deiodinase and uncoupling protein in brown adipose tissue of human newborns." *J Clin Endocrinol Metab* **77**(2), 382–387.

Houstek, J., Kopecky, J., Rychter, Z., and Soukup, T. (1988). "Uncoupling protein in embryonic brown adipose tissue – existence of nonthermogenic and thermogenic mitochondria." *Biochim Biophys Acta* **935**(1), 19–25.

Knip, M. and Akerblom, H. K. (2005). "Early nutrition and later diabetes risk." *Adv Exp Med Biol* **569**, 142–150.

Korotkova, M., Gabrielsson, B., Lonn, M., Hanson, L. A., and Strandvik, B. (2002). "Leptin levels in rat offspring are modified by the ratio of linoleic to alpha-linolenic acid in the maternal diet." *J Lipid Res* **43**(10), 1743–1749.

Kunesova, M., Braunerova, R., Hlavaty, P., Tvrzicka, E., Stankova, B., Skrha, J., Hilgertova, J., Hill, M., Kopecky, J., Wagenknecht, M., Hainer, V., Matoulek, M., Parizkova, J., Zak, A., and Svacina, S. (2006). "The influence of n-3 polyunsaturated fatty acids and very low calorie diet during a short-term weight reducing regimen on weight loss and serum fatty acid composition in severely obese women." *Physiol Res* **55**(1), 63–72.

Lillycrop, K. A., Phillips, E. S., Jackson, A. A., Hanson, M. A., and Burdge, G. C. (2005). "Dietary protein restriction of pregnant rats induces and folic acid supplementation prevents epigenetic modification of hepatic gene expression in the offspring." *J Nutr* **135**(6), 1382–1386.

Lombardo, Y. B. and Chicco, A. G. (2006). "Effects of dietary polyunsaturated n-3 fatty acids on dyslipidemia and insulin resistance in rodents and humans. A review." *J Nutr Biochem* **17**(1), 1–13.

Mace, K., Shahkhalili, Y., Aprikian, O., and Stan, S. (2006). "Dietary fat and fat types as early determinants of childhood obesity: a reappraisal." *Int J Obes (Lond)* **30**(Suppl 4), S50–S57.

Madsen, L., Petersen, R. K., and Kristiansen, K. (2005). "Regulation of adipocyte differentiation and function by polyunsaturated fatty acids." *Biochim Biophys Acta* **1740**(2), 266–286.

Massiera, F., Saint-Marc, P., Seydoux, J., Murata, T., Kobayashi, T., Narumiya, S., Guesnet, P., Amri, E. Z., Negrel, R., and Ailhaud, G. (2003). "Arachidonic acid and prostacyclin signaling promote adipose tissue development: a human health concern?" *J Lipid Res* **44**(2), 271–279.

Merklin, R. J. (1974). "Growth and distribution of human fetal brown fat." *Anat Rec* **178**(3), 637–645.

Minokoshi, Y., Kim, Y. B., Peroni, O. D., Fryer, L. G., Muller, C., Carling, D., and Kahn, B. B. (2002). "Leptin stimulates fatty-acid oxidation by activating AMP-activated protein kinase." *Nature* **415**(6869), 339–343.

Miralles, O., Sanchez, J., Palou, A., and Pico, C. (2006). "A physiological role of breast milk leptin in body weight control in developing infants." *Obesity (Silver Spring)* **14**(8), 1371–1377.

Ruxton, C. H., Reed, S. C., Simpson Double Dagger, M. J., and Millington, K. J. (2004). "The health benefits of omega-3 polyunsaturated fatty acids: a review of the evidence." *J Hum Nutr Diet* **17**(5), 449–459.

Ruzickova, J., Rossmeisl, M., Prazak, T., Flachs, P., Sponarova, J., Vecka, M., Tvrzicka, E., Bryhn, M., and Kopecky, J. (2004). "Omega-3 PUFA of marine origin limit diet-induced obesity in mice by reducing cellularity of adipose tissue." *Lipids* **39**(12), 1177–1185.

Serhan, C. N. (2005). "Novel omega – 3-derived local mediators in anti-inflammation and resolution." *Pharmacol Ther* **105**(1), 7–21.

Sevillano, J., Lopez-Perez, I. C., Herrera, E., Del Pilar, R. M., and Bocos, C. (2005). "Englitazone administration to late pregnant rats produces delayed body growth and insulin resistance in their fetuses and neonates." *Biochem J* **389**(Pt 3), 913–918.

Siemelink, M., Verhoef, A., Dormans, J. A., Span, P. N., and Piersma, A. H. (2002). "Dietary fatty acid composition during pregnancy and lactation in the rat programs growth and glucose metabolism in the offspring." *Diabetologia* **45**(10), 1397–1403.

Stocker, C. J., Wargent, E., O'Dowd, J., Cornick, C., Speakman, J. R., Arch, J. R., and Cawthorne, M. A. (2007). "Prevention of diet-induced obesity and impaired glucose tolerance in rats following administration of leptin to their mothers." *AJP – Regul Integ Comp Physiol* **292**(5), R1810–R1818.

Storlien, L. H., Kraegen, E. W., Chisholm, D. J., Ford, G. L., Bruce, D. G., and Pascoe, W. S. (1987). "Fish oil prevents insulin resistance induced by high-fat feeding in rats." *Science* **237**(4817), 885–888.

Storlien, L. H., Jenkins, A. B., Chisholm, D. J., Pascoe, W. S., Khouri, S., and Kraegen, E. W. (1991). "Influence of dietary fat composition on development of insulin resistance in rats. Relationship to muscle triglyceride and omega-3 fatty acids in muscle phospholipid." *Diabetes* **40**(2), 280–289.

Uauy, R., Hoffman, D. R., Mena, P., Llanos, A., and Birch, E. E. (2003). "Term infant studies of DHA and ARA supplementation on neurodevelopment: results of randomized controlled trials." *J Pediatr* **143**(Suppl 4), S17–S25.

Waterland, R. A. and Rached, M.-T. (2006). "Developmental establishment of epigenotype: a role for dietary fatty acids?" *Scand J Food Nutr* **50**(Suppl 2), 21–26.

Yamauchi, T., Kamon, J., Minokoshi, Y., Ito, Y., Waki, H., Uchida, S., Yamashita, S., Noda, M., Kita, S., Ueki, K., Eto, K., Akanuma, Y., Froguel, P., Foufelle, F., Ferre, P., Carling, D., Kimura, S., Nagai, R., Kahn, B. B., and Kadowaki, T. (2002). "Adiponectin stimulates glucose utilization and fatty-acid oxidation by activating AMP-activated protein kinase." *Nat Med* **8**(11), 1288–1295.

Yura, S., Itoh, H., Sagawa, N., Yamamoto, H., Masuzaki, H., Nakao, K., Kawamura, M., Takemura, M., Kakui, K., Ogawa, Y., and Fujii, S. (2005). "Role of premature leptin surge in obesity resulting from intrauterine undernutrition." *Cell Metab* **1**(6), 371–378.

Trans Isomeric and LCPUFA Are Inversely Correlated in Erythrocyte Membrane Lipids at Mid-gestation

Tamás Marosvölgyi, Cristina Campoy, Berthold Koletzko, Éva Szabó, Viktoria Jakobik, Margarita Jimenez, Hans Demmelmair, and Tamás Decsi

Abstract Fatty acid composition of erythrocyte phosphatidylcholines was determined by high-resolution capillary gas chromatography in Spanish (n = 120), German (n = 78) and Hungarian (n = 43) expectant women at the 20th week of gestation. The sum of *trans* isomeric fatty acids was significantly ($p < 0.05$) lower in Hungarian (0.68 [0.43]% wt/wt, median [IQR]) than in Spanish (0.82 [0.53]) expectant women. There were no significant correlations between the sum of *trans* isomers and linoleic acid or alpha-linolenic acid in either of the three groups. In contrast, there were significant inverse correlations between the sum of *trans* fatty acids and arachidonic acid and docosahexaenoic acid in all the three groups. These data raise the possibility that maternal *trans* isomeric fatty acid status may be inversely associated to the essential fatty acid status of the foetus.

Keywords Arachidonic acid • docosahexaenoic acid • foetal nutrition • *trans* fatty acids

Abbreviations AA: arachidonic acid; ALA: alpha-linolenic acid; DHA: docosahexaenoic acid; LA: linoleic acid; LCPUFA: long-chain polyunsaturated fatty acid; C18:1*t*: *trans* hexadecenoic acid

1 Introduction

Unsaturated fatty acids are usually found in nature in their *cis* configuration form, while *trans* isomers are produced in the rumen of ruminant animals and during the hydrogenation of oils. *Cis* double bonds break the spatial linearity of the

T. Marosvölgyi, É. Szabó, V. Jakobik, and T. Decsi (✉)
Department of Paediatrics, University of Pécs, Pécs, Hungary
tamas.decsi@aok.pte.hu

C. Campoy and M. Jimenez
Department of Paediatrics, University of Granada, Granada, Spain

B. Koletzko and H. Demmelmair
Dr. von Haunersches Kinderspital, University of Munich, Munich, Germany

B. Koletzko et al. (eds.), *Early Nutrition Programming and Health Outcomes in Later Life: Obesity and Beyond*,

carbon chain, while *trans* fatty acids, similarly to saturated fatty acids, are linear in space; the different biological properties of the *cis* and the *trans* isomers of the same unsaturated fatty acids arise mainly from the different spatial configuration (Koletzko and Decsi 1997). Because *cis* and *trans* isomeric fatty acids use the same enzymes during their metabolism, *trans* fatty acids may disturb the desaturation and chain elongation of essential fatty acids, the n-6 linoleic acid (LA; C18:2n-6) and the n-3 alpha-linolenic acid (ALA; C18:3n-3) to their respective LCPUFA metabolites, arachidonic acid (AA; C20:4n-6) and docosahexanoic acid (DHA; C22:6n-3). The most important n-3 LCPUFA, DHA plays an important role in the early development of central nervous system; hence, optimal perinatal DHA supply is of great concern. Previously we found significant inverse correlations between *trans* isomers and LCPUFAs in cord blood lipids of preterm (Koletzko 1992) and full-term infants (Decsi et al. 2001) as well as in mature human milk samples (Szabó et al. 2007). Here we report data on the association of the availability of *trans* fatty acids to those of LCPUFA in maternal blood lipids at mid gestation.

2 Methods

At the 20th week of gestation we collected blood samples of German (n = 78), Hungarian (n = 43) and Spanish (n = 120) expectant women participating in the NUHEAL study. Detailed description of the supplementation study has been provided elsewhere (Decsi et al. 2005; Krauss-Etschman et al. 2007). Briefly, apparently healthy pregnant women were recruited before the 20th week of gestation in the Departments of Obstetrics at Ludwig Maximilians University, Munich, Germany; the University of Granada, Granada, Spain; and the University of Pécs, Pécs, Hungary. Inclusion criteria were singleton pregnancy, gestational age lower than 20 weeks at enrolment, and intention to deliver in one of the obstetrical centres. Women with serious chronic illness or those using fish oil supplements since the beginning of pregnancy or folate or vitamin B_{12} supplements after the 16th week of gestation were excluded from the study.

Fatty acid composition of erythrocyte membrane lipids was determined by high-resolution gas–liquid chromatography. Statistical analysis was performed with the use of SPSS 11.5 for Windows. Differences between the three nations were calculated with the analysis of variance followed by Mann-Whitney test, whereas correlations between fatty acids were calculated with Spearman's rho correlation analysis. In this paper, we focus on phosphatidylcholines.

3 Results

Values of *trans* hexadecenoic acid (C16:1*t*) were significantly higher in German (0.20 [0.16], % wt/wt, median [IQR]) than in Spanish (0.16 [0.16], $p < 0.05$) and Hungarian mothers (0.14 [0.12], $p < 0.05$). There were no significant differences in

Table 1 Spearman's rho correlation coefficients for n-6 and n-3 polyunsaturated fatty acids in erythrocyte membrane phosphatidylcholines in European expectant women at the 20th week of gestation

C18:1*t*	Spanish (n = 120)	German (n = 78)	Hungarian (n = 43)
LA	−0.113	−0.158	0.062
AA	−0.287[a]	−0.706[b]	−0.446[a]
ALA	−0.025	0.061	0.058
DHA	−0.431[b]	−0.733[b]	−0.342[c]

For abbreviations, see list of abbreviations in text.
[a]$p < 0.01$.
[b]$p < 0.001$.
[c]$p < 0.05$.

trans octadecenoic acid (C18:1*t*) values, whereas values of *trans* octadecadienoic acid (C18:2*tt*) were significantly lower in Hungarian (0.10 [0.12]) than in Spanish (0.18 [0.15], $p < 0.01$) and German (0.16 [0.19], $p < 0.05$) mothers. The sum of *trans* fatty acids was significantly higher in Spanish (0.82 [0.53]) than in Hungarian mothers (0.68 [0.43], $p < 0.05$).

There was no significant correlation between C18:1*t* and the parent essential fatty acids, LA and ALA (Table 1). In contrast, we found significant inverse correlations between 18:1*t* and the most important n-6 metabolite, AA and in all three groups European expecting women (Table 1). Similarly, the values of 18:1*t* and the most important n-3 metabolite, DHA were found to be in significant inverse correlation in all the three nations (Table 1).

4 Discussion

Although human metabolism is able to elongate and desaturate ingested *trans* isomeric fatty acids into longer-chain and more unsaturated metabolites, it is unable to *de novo* synthesize *trans* fatty acids. Hence, *trans* fatty acids detected in blood lipids of expectant women must originate from their diet. In the present study, we found significant inverse correlations between *trans* isomeric fatty acids and n-3 and n-6 LCPUFAs in erythrocyte membrane phosphatidylcholines at the 20th week of gestation in German and Hungarian and Spanish women. To the best of our knowledge, this is the first report indicating untoward effects of dietary *trans* fatty acid intakes on the availability of LCPUFA in expecting women.

However, the present study is not the first one reporting inverse relationship between *trans* fatty acids and LCPUFAs in the perinatal period. Significant inverse correlations were found between *trans* isomeric fatty acids and LCPUFAs in cord blood lipids both in healthy full-term infants (Elias and Innis 2001) and in full-term infants with an atopic trait (Decsi et al. 2001), in cord vessel wall lipids in healthy full-term infants (Decsi et al. 2002) and in plasma lipids in young preterm infants

(Koletzko 1992). Moreover, recent data indicate that *trans* fatty acids may be inversely related not only to LCPUFA status, but to results of neurodevelopmental tests as well. The study, determining relationships between relative fatty acid contents of umbilical arteries and veins and neurodevelopment at 18 months, comprised a mixed group of 317 healthy, full-term infants fed human milk and formula with or without preformed dietary LCPUFA (Bouwstra et al. 2006). Study endpoints were the Hempel neurological examination resulting in a neurological classification and neurological optimality score, and the Bayley Psychomotor and Mental Developmental Indices. Umbilical vein AA values were related to neurological optimality score in univariate statistics but not in multivariate analyses. However, the sum of *trans* fatty acids and that of trans fatty acids with 18 carbon atoms showed a negative association with neurological optimality score in both univariate and multivariate analyses.

5 Conclusions

In summary, the results obtained in the present study indicate that maternal *trans* isomeric fatty acids may have an adverse effect on the availability of LCPUFAs. The recent observation that high *trans* fatty acid contents in umbilical vein wall lipids were related to poorer performances in neurological tests at the age of 18 months (Bouwstra et al. 2006) underpins the potential relevance of reducing maternal trans fatty acid intakes during pregnancy.

References

Bouwstra, H., J. Dijck-Brouwer, T. Decsi, G. Boehm, E.R. Boersma, F.A. Muskiet, M. Hadders-Algra (2006) "Neurologic condition of healthy term infants at 18 months: positive association with venous umbilical DHA status and negative association with umbilical trans-fatty acids." *Pediatr Res* **60(3)**:334–339.

Decsi, T., I. Burus, S. Molnár, H. Minda, V. Veitl (2001) "Inverse association between trans isomeric and long-chain polyunsaturated fatty acids in cord blood lipids of full-term infants." *Am J Clin Nutr* **74(3)**:364–368.

Decsi, T., G. Boehm, H.M.R. Tjoonk, S. Molnár, D.A. Dijck-Brouwer, M. Hadders-Algra, I.A. Martini, F.A. Muskiet, E.R. Boersma (2002) "*Trans* isomeric octadecenoic acids are related inversely to arachidonic acid and DHA and positively to mead acid in umbilical vessel wall lipids." *Lipids* **37**:959–965.

Decsi, T., C. Campoy, B. Koletzko (2005) "Effect of n-3 polyunsaturated fatty acid supplementation in pregnancy: the NUHEAL trial." *Adv Exp Med Biol* **569**:109–113.

Elias, S.L., S.M. Innis (2001) "Infant plasma *trans*, n-6, and n-3 fatty acids and conjugated linoleic acids are related to maternal plasma fatty acids, length of gestation, and birth weight and length." *Am J Clin Nutr* **73**:807–814.

Koletzko, B. (1992) "*Trans* fatty acids may impair biosynthesis of long-chain polyunsaturates and growth in man." *Acta Paediatr Scand* **81**:302–306.

Koletzko, B., T. Decsi (1997) "Metabolic aspects of *trans* fatty acids." *Clin Nutr* **16**:229–237.

Krauss-Etschmann, S., R. Shadid, C. Campoy, E. Hoster, H. Demmelmair, M. Jiménez, A. Gil, M. Rivero, B. Veszprémi, T. Decsi, B.V. Koletzko, Nutrition and Health Lifestyle (NUHEAL) Study Group (2007) "Effects of fish-oil and folate supplementation of pregnant women on maternal and fetal plasma concentrations of docosahexaenoic acid and eicosapentaenoic acid: a European randomized multicenter trial." *Am J Clin Nutr* **85**:1392–1400.

Szabó, É., G. Boehm, C. Beermann, M. Weyermann, H. Brenner, D. Rothenbacher, T. Decsi (2007) "Trans octadecenoic acid and trans octadecadienoic acid are inversely related to long-chain polyunsaturates in human milk: results of a large birth cohort study." *Am J Clin Nutr* **85**(5):1320–1327.

Early Growth and Body Composition in Infancy

Sirinuch Chomtho, Jonathan C.K. Wells, Peter S. Davies, Alan Lucas, and Mary S. Fewtrell

Abstract Examination of the relationship between early growth and body composition (BC) in infancy might provide clues about the mechanism of early nutrition programming. 150 healthy full-term infants (64 boys) born in Cambridge from 1985–1993 had BC measured using stable isotope at the age of 12 weeks as a part of infant nutrition studies. Fat mass index (FMI, FM/length^2) and lean mass index (LMI, LM/length^2) internal standard deviation scores (SDS) were calculated for boys and girls. Birth weight SDS was positively associated with length, BMI and FMI SDS at 12 weeks, but not LMI SDS; equivalent to 0.26 SDS increase in FMI per 1 SDS increase in birth weight (95% CI, 0.04–0.48). Weight SDS change from birth-12 weeks was positively correlated with FMI and LMI SDS at 12 weeks; equivalent to 0.68 SDS and 0.48 SDS increase in FMI and LMI per 1 SDS gain in weight (95% CI, 0.48–0.88 and 0.26–0.70, respectively). Associations were independent of gender, parity, infant diets, and, for weight gain, birth weight SDS. Conclusion: Higher birth weight was associated with higher fat mass at 3 months whereas rapid weight gain in the first 3 months was associated with both fat and lean mass. Our data do not support the hypothesis that lean mass tracks directly from fetal life to childhood.

Keywords Body composition • growth • infant nutrition • programming

Abbreviations BC: body composition; FM: fat mass; FMI: fat mass index; LM: lean mass; LMI: lean mass index; SDS: standard deviation score; TBW: total body water; Δ weight SDS: change in weight SDS; Δ length SDS: change in length SDS

S. Chomtho (✉), J.C.K. Wells, A. Lucas, and M.S. Fewtrell
MRC Childhood Nutrition Research Centre, Institute of Child Health, University College London
s.chomtho@ich.ucl.ac.uk

P.S. Davies
Children's Nutrition Research Centre, Discipline of Paediatrics and Child Health, University of Queensland

B. Koletzko et al. (eds.), *Early Nutrition Programming and Health Outcomes in Later Life: Obesity and Beyond*,

1 Introduction

The concept that events operating in early life influence or 'programme' (Lucas 1991) later health has been extensively investigated in the last 2 decades. Studies in rodents and primates suggest that infant overnutrition and excessive weight gain are predisposing factors for obesity in later life even when early dietary effects are transitory (Aubert et al. 1980; Lewis et al. 1989). Recent studies in humans have consistently found positive associations between birth weight and later lean body mass, while data from longitudinal studies suggest that rapid infancy weight gain is associated with higher BMI, with the effects on body composition (BC) varying by population, i.e. relating with higher lean mass (LM) in developing countries, but predicting subsequent fat mass (FM) in western populations (see the recent review in *Proceedings of the Nutrition Society*) (Wells et al. 2007). Examination of the relationship between early growth and BC in infancy might provide clues about the mechanism of early nutrition programming.

2 Methods

We studied 150 healthy full-term infants (64 boys) who were born in Cambridge from 1985–1993 and had BC measured using stable isotope at the age of 12 weeks as a part of infant nutrition studies. Total body water (TBW) was measured by oral administration of a dose of 0.1 g per kg body weight of water labelled with ^{2}H. The $^{2}H_2O$ enrichment in a urine sample was used to calculate TBW (from the principle of dilution after equilibration of this dose with body water pool was complete) (Davies and Wells 1994). Infant BC was then calculated assuming a certain hydration fraction of LM in infancy (Fomon et al. 1982). FM was calculated from the difference between body weight and LM. Fat mass index (FMI, FM/length^2) and lean mass index (LMI, LM/length^2) internal standard deviation score (SDS) were calculated for boys and girls. Weight, length, and BMI SDS were calculated using the British 1990 reference (Cole et al. 1998). Multiple linear regression was used to assess the associations between early growth parameters and infant BC adjusting for potential confounders.

3 Results

There was no difference in birth weight SDS and 12 weeks BMI SDS for this dataset compared to the British 1990 reference (data not shown). From Table 1, birth weight SDS was positively associated with length, BMI and FMI SDS at 12 weeks, but not LMI SDS; equivalent to 0.26 SDS increase in FMI per 1 SDS

Table 1 Association of birth weight SDS and infant BC at 12 weeks

	B	SE	p	r^2
Length SDS	0.58	0.07	**<0.001**	0.25
BMI SDS	0.29	0.09	**0.001**	0.05
FMI SDS	0.26	0.11	**0.02**	0.04
LMI SDS	0.07	0.11	0.55	

Each row represents a different model with infant BC in the left hand column as a dependent variable; birth weight SDS was an independent variable; exact age, gender, parity, and infant diets were covariates; B = the coefficient of birth weight SDS i.e. the change in body composition per 1 SDS increase in birth weight, SE = standard error, bold p values indicate significant at $p < 0.05$, r^2 = the proportion of variability in BC SDS explained by birth weight SDS.

increase in birth weight (95% CI, 0.04–0.48). Birth length SDS (n = 58) showed a positive association with LM at 12 weeks; however, the association was attenuated substantively and become non-significant after adjusting for length using LMI (data not shown).

From Table 2, change in weight SDS (Δ weight SDS) from birth-12 weeks was positively correlated with FMI and LMI SDS at 12 weeks; equivalent to 0.68 SDS and 0.48 SDS increase in FMI and LMI per 1 SDS gain in weight (95% CI, 0.48–0.88 and 0.26–0.70, respectively). Associations were independent of gender, parity, infant diets, and birth weight SDS. Change in length SDS (Δ length SDS) during the same period was not associated with any measurement at 12 weeks other than length SDS. There was no significant interaction between birth SDS and Δ weight SDS in predicting infant BC. Variability in infant BC at 3 months was explained more by Δ weight SDS than by birth weight SDS.

Table 2 Association of weight and length SDS change from birth to 12 weeks with body composition

	Δ Weight SDS (n = 150)				Δ Length SDS (n = 58)			
	B	SE	p	r^2	B	SE	p	r^2
Length SDS	0.49	0.07	**<0.001**	0.22	0.71	0.09	**<0.001**	0.43
BMI SDS	0.99	0.06	**<0.001**	0.62	0.17	0.14	0.23	
FMI SDS	0.68	0.10	**<0.001**	0.23	0.08	0.20	0.69	
LMI SDS	0.48	0.11	**<0.001**	0.12	0.09	0.20	0.65	

Each row represents a different model with infant BC in the left hand column as a dependent variable; either Δ weight SDS or Δ length SDS was an independent variable; exact age, gender, parity, infant diets, and birth weight SDS were covariates; B = the change in body composition per 1 SDS increase in Δ weight or Δ length, SE = standard error, bold p value indicate significant at $p < 0.05$, r^2 = the proportion of variability in BC SDS explained by Δ weight SDS or Δ length SDS.

4 Discussion

An important question is whether the association between early 'growth' (generally early weight gain) and later BC is mediated through 'structural' changes in infant BC which then track through adolescent and adult life, or through some other mechanism that does not involve infant BC. If the latter is true, weight gain might be regarded as essentially an 'epiphenomenon'. We have shown that higher birth weight was associated with higher FM at 3 months whereas rapid weight gain in the first 3 months was associated with both higher rank of fat and lean mass. From our data, the evidence implicating infant BC in the programming process was not strong; they do not support the hypothesis that lean mass tracks directly from fetal life to childhood. However, we cannot exclude the possibility that the critical period for any programming effects of infant BC is earlier than 12 weeks. The other possibility, not tested in our study, is that early infant growth programs later BC by changing some 'functional' component(s) that in turn regulate the subsequent development of fatness. Likely candidates include the set-point of hormones regulating growth or appetite such as insulin, IGF-1, or leptin (Cripps et al. 2005; McMillen et al. 2004; Remacle et al. 2004). Such effects could persist and explain the observed long-term influence on later BC and risk of obesity.

References

Aubert, R., Suquet, J.P., and Lemonnier, D. (1980) Long-term morphological and metabolic effects of early under- and over-nutrition in mice. *J Nutr* **110**: 649–661.

Cole, T.J., Freeman, J.V., and Preece, M.A. (1998) British 1990 growth reference centiles for weight, height, body mass index and head circumference fitted by maximum penalized likelihood. *Stat Med* **17**: 407–429.

Cripps, R.L., Martin-Gronert, M.S., and Ozanne, S.E. (2005) Fetal and perinatal programming of appetite. *Clin Sci (Lond)* **109**: 1–11.

Davies, P.S. and Wells, J.C. (1994) Calculation of total body water in infancy. *Eur J Clin Nutr* **48**: 490–495.

Fomon, S.J., Haschke, F., Ziegler, E.E., and Nelson, S.E. (1982) Body composition of reference children from birth to age 10 years. *Am J Clin Nutr* **35**: 1169–1175.

Lewis, D.S., Bertrand, H.A., McMahan, C.A., McGill, H.C., Jr., Carey, K.D., and Masoro, E.J. (1989) Influence of preweaning food intake on body composition of young adult baboons. *Am J Physiol* **257**: R1128–R1135.

Lucas, A. (1991) Programming by early nutrition in man. In *The childhood environment and adult disease*, Bock, G.R. and Whelan, J. (eds.). Chichester: Wiley, pp. 38–55.

McMillen, I.C., Muhlhausler, B.S., Duffield, J.A., and Yuen, B.S. (2004) Prenatal programming of postnatal obesity: fetal nutrition and the regulation of leptin synthesis and secretion before birth. *Proc Nutr Soc* **63**: 405–412.

Remacle, C., Bieswal, F., and Reusens, B. (2004) Programming of obesity and cardiovascular disease. *Int J Obes Relat Metab Disord* **28**(Suppl 3): S46–S53.

Wells, J.C.K., Chomtho, S., and Fewtrell, M.S. (2007) Programming of body composition by early growth and nutrition. *Proc Nutr Soc* **66**: 423–434.

Obesity Related Programming Statements in Infant Feeding Policies in Five European Countries

Elena Martin-Bautista, Cristina Campoy, Tamás Decsi, Szilvia Bokor, Julia von Rosen-von Hoewel, Kirsi Laitinen, Martina A. Schmid, Jane Morgan, Heather Gage, Berthold Koletzko, and Monique Raats

Abstract The aim of this study was to know how the early nutrition programming concept and its relation with long-term diseases such as obesity is reflected in policy recommendations on infant nutrition in five European countries (Finland, Germany, Hungary, Spain and England). After collating and evaluating infant nutrition policy documents, statements about early nutrition programming, as the origin of diseases such as obesity, were analysed. The number of policy documents analysed were 38 (England: 10, Finland: 2, Germany: 11, Hungary: 8, Spain: 7) with a total of 455 statements identified and categorized into 53 different health outcomes. Obesity was mentioned in 5.5% (n = 25) of the statements, the third most frequent outcome after allergy (14.1%, n = 64) and health in general (5.7%, n = 26). Twenty six percent (n = 6) of the obesity related statements referred to short-term duration of the effects, 48% (n = 12) to medium-term, 24% (n = 6) to long-term effects and the rest were not identified. Only 22% of the obesity statements were evidence based. The link between infant feeding and obesity is integrated into policy documents, but most of the statements did not fully specify the short, medium and long term health implications. Action may be required to keep documents up to date as new evidence emerges and to ensure the evidence base is properly recorded.

E. Martin-Bautista and C. Campoy (✉)
Department of Paediatrics, University of Granada, Spain
ccampoy@ugr.es

T. Decsi and S. Bokor
Department of Paediatrics, University of Pécs, Hungary

K. Laitinen
Department of Paediatrics, University of Turku, Finland

J. von Rosen-von Hoewel and B. Koletzko
Dr. von Hauner Children's Hospital, Ludwig-Maximilians University, Munich, Germany

M.A. Schmid, J. Morgan, H. Gage, and M. Raats
Food, Consumer Behaviour and Health Research Centre, University of Surrey, Guildford, UK

B. Koletzko et al. (eds.), *Early Nutrition Programming and Health Outcomes in Later Life: Obesity and Beyond*,

Keywords Early nutrition programming • European Union • obesity • policies

Abbreviations BF: breastfeeding; RCT: randomized controlled trial; WHO: World Health Organization

1 Introduction

Evidence is accumulating that the nutrition of women during pregnancy (Decsi et al. 2005), breastfeeding (BF) (Koletzko 2006) and complementary feeding of infants can have implications for child development and long-term health (Lucas 2005; Demmelmair et al. 2006). In certain circumstances the early nutrition environment may alter or 'programme' a baby's metabolism in a way that increases the risks of disease later in life (Lucas 1991, 1994). Programming has been linked to a range of short, medium and long term health outcomes including obesity. The World Health Organization (WHO) considers obesity to be one of the most serious chronic diseases (WHO 2002). The current prevalence of obesity has already reached unprecedented levels and the rate at which it is annually increasing in most developed regions is substantial (Brug 2007; Kelishadi 2007). This study presents an overview of the information reflected about early nutrition programming in relation to long-term diseases, such as obesity, in infant nutrition policy documents in five member states of the European Union.

2 Material and Methods

A search for current publicly available national policy documents was carried out from July to October 2005 within five European countries: England, Finland, Germany, Hungary and Spain. All recommendations or guidelines about breastfeeding, introduction of solid foods and beverages and infant feeding in the first year of life were included. The documents were screened for statements on the relationship between infant feeding and health outcomes. Particular emphasis was placed on coverage of the relationship between early nutrition and obesity. Statements were translated into English by local researchers and classified according to: the nutrition behaviour each referred to (BF in general, exclusively BF for 4 or 6 months and complementary feeding); the health outcome for the offspring (for example, obesity, infections, diabetes, allergy, cardiovascular disease, cancer, etc.); the duration of this health outcome (short – to 5 years, medium – 5–15 years, or long term – more than 15 years). The evidence and citations used in the statements were recorded and categorized according to the Cochrane Library type of strength of evidence. Data were entered into SPSS version 14.0 (SPSS Chicago, IL, USA) and descriptive statistical analysis was undertaken.

3 Results

The number of policy documents analysed was 38 (England: 10, Finland: 2, Germany: 11, Hungary: 8, Spain: 7) with a total of 455 statements identified and categorized into 53 different health outcomes. Of the total statements, 184 (40.4%) concerned the effect of BF in general, 47 (10.3%) emphasized the exclusivity of BF and 34 (7.5%) targeted the introduction of complementary food. Only 24 (5.3%) of the statements mentioned the potential long-term benefits of exclusive BF in the first 6 months of life.

Most statements n = 269 (59.1%) were not supported by reference to evidence. Where the evidence base was cited, 39.2% were expert committees, 23.1% were non randomized trials, 14.5% were randomized controlled trials (RCTs), 13.4% were uncontrolled observational studies and 3.2% were reviews of RCTs. In the case of obesity, only 22% of the statements had evidence supporting them. This disease was mentioned in n = 25 (5.5%) of the statements, and was the third most frequently reported outcome after allergy (14.1%, n = 64) and health in general (5.7%, n = 26). Obesity was ranked differently among countries, being the second most frequently cited health outcome in Hungary, fourth in Germany and Spain and ninth in England and Finland. 26% (n = 6) of the obesity related statements referred to short-term duration of the effects, 48% (n = 12) to medium-term, 24% (n = 6) to long-term effects and the rest were not identified.

4 Discussion

This review of current policy documents of five EU countries found that they contained many statements that linked infant feeding to health outcomes. The concept of early nutrition programming purports that diet in the first stages of life is important in the development of diseases in later life (Lucas 2005) such as diabetes (Steyn et al. 2004), cardiovascular diseases (Reddy and Katan 2004), certain types of cancer (Key et al. 2004) and for neurological development (Dijck-Brouwer et al. 2005). The WHO aims to avoid a pandemic of chronic disease (WHO 2003) and is conscious of early life nutritional influences on the genesis of non-transmissible diseases in later adult life (Yach et al. 2004). Programming effects may be triggered by the intra uterine nutritional environment as well as in the perinatal period. This paper shows that obesity is featured highly amongst outcomes covered in the policy documents of the study countries. Many studies have been published recently regarding the potential protective effect of breast-feeding on childhood obesity (Koletzko 2006). There is increasingly strong evidence suggesting that a lower risk of developing obesity (Gillman et al. 2001; von Kries et al. 1999) may be directly related to duration of exclusive BF although the effects may not become evident until later in childhood. Promoting BF has many benefits, the prevention of childhood obesity probably being one of them. But, only 5.3% of identified statements mentioned the potential effects of exclusively BF for 6 months, whereas 40.4% only talked about BF in general, without specification. More than half of the statements that were identified in policy documents were not linked to evidence, and, in the case of obesity, only 22% of them were. The absence of evidence is perhaps surprising as policy documents that fully show the rationale for their recommendations and the basis for statements may carry more credibility and be more effective in promoting appropriate infant nutrition behaviour.

5 Conclusions

In summary, the link between infant feeding and obesity is integrated into policy documents, but most of the statements did not fully specify the short, medium and long term health implications. Moreover, action may be required to keep documents up to date as new evidence emerges and to ensure the evidence base is properly recorded.

Acknowledgments This study was supported as a part of the European Project "Early Nutrition Programming-EARNEST" within the sixth Framework Programme. N° FOOD-CT-2005-007036.

References

Brug J (2007, Apr 5). The European charter for counteracting obesity: a late but important step towards action. Observations on the WHO-Europe ministerial conference. Istanbul, November 15–17, 2006. *Int J Behav Nutr Phys Act* **4**:11.

Decsi T, Campoy C, Koletzko B (2005). Effect of N-3 polyunsaturated fatty acid supplementation in pregnancy: the Nuheal trial. *Adv Exp Med Biol* **569**:109–113

Demmelmair H, von Rosen J, Koletzko B (2006, Aug). Long-term consequences of early nutrition. *Early Hum Dev* **82**(8):567–574.

Dijck-Brouwer DA, Hadders-Algra M, Bouwstra H, Decsi T, Boehm G, Martini IA, Boersma ER, Muskiet FA (2005, Jan). Lower fetal status of docosahexaenoic acid, arachidonic acid and essential fatty acids is associated with less favorable neonatal neurological condition. *Prostaglandins Leukot Essent Fatty Acids* **72**(1):21–28.

Gillman MW et al. (2001). Risk of overweight among adolescents who were breastfed as infants. *J Am Med Assoc* **285**:2461–2467.

Kelishadi R (2007, May 3). Childhood overweight, obesity, and the metabolic syndrome in developing countries. *Epidemiol Rev* (Epub ahead of print).

Key YJ, Schatzkin A, Willett WC, Allen NE, Spencer EA, Travis RC (2004). Diet, nutrition and the prevention of cancer. *Public Health Nutr* **7**(1A):187–200.

Koletzko B (2006). Long-term consequences of early feeding on later obesity risk. *Nestle Nutr Workshop Ser Pediatr Prog* **58**:1–18.

Lucas A (1991). Programming by early nutrition in man. In: Bock GR, Whelan J (eds.), *The childhood environment and adult disease* (*CIBA Foundation Symposium 156*). Chichester: Wiley, pp. 38–55.

Lucas A (1994, Oct). Role of nutritional programming in determining adult morbidity. *Arch Dis Child* **71**(4):288–290.

Lucas A (2005, May). Long-term programming effects of early nutrition – implications for the preterm infant. *J Perinatol* **25**(Suppl 2):S2–S6.
Reddy KS, Katan MB (2004). Diet, nutrition and the prevention of hypertension and cardiovascular diseases. *Public Health Nutr* **7**(1A):167–186.
Steyn NP, Mann J, Bennet PH, Temple N, Zimmel P, Tuomilehto J, et al. (2004). Diet, nutrition and the prevention of type 2 diabetes. *Public Health Nutr* **7**(1A):147–165.
von Kries, Koletzko B, Sauerwald T, von ME, Barnert D, Grunert V, von Voss H (1999, Jul 17). Breast feeding and obesity: cross sectional study. *BMJ* **319**(7203):147–150.
WHO – World Health Organization Expert Consultation (2002). The optimal duration of exclusive breastfeeding. Geneva, Switzerland: World Health Organization.
WHO – World Health Organization. Report of the Joint WHO/FAO Expert (2003). Consultation on diet, nutrition and prevention of chronic diseases. WHO Technical Report Series 916.
Yach D, Hawkes C, Gould CL and Hofman KJ (2004). 'The global burden of chronic diseases: overcoming impediments to prevention and control (Special Communication).' *JAMA* **291**:2616–2622.

Obesity Related Programming Statements in Materials on Infant Feeding Aimed at Parents in Five European Countries

Julia von Rosen-von Hoewel, Kirsi Laitinen, Elena Martin-Bautista, Cristina Campoy, Viktoria Jakobik, Tamás Decsi, Martina A. Schmid, Jane Morgan, Heather Gage, Berthold Koletzko, and Monique Raats

Abstract Early nutrition programming as an origin of obesity is well acknowledged, but to what extent is this concept communicated to parents? In five European countries, UK, Finland (FI), Germany (DE), Hungary (HU) and Spain (ES), a total of 130 stand alone leaflets and 161 articles from parenting magazines providing information on feeding of healthy infants aged 0–12 months were identified and screened for nutrition programming statements. Obesity was mentioned in 8.5% (54/638) of the statements, and was the fourth most frequent outcome after allergy (20.7%), risk of infections (15.5%) and growth and development (11.4%). A temporal prognosis was given in 39% of obesity related statements, 6% referring to short- (<5 years), 13% to medium- (5–15 years) and 20% to long-term (>15 years) duration of effects. So advice on obesity focuses on the intrinsic long-term perspective of programming in contrary to other surveyed health-outcomes where only 8% considered a lifelong approach. The major programming related behaviour concerned breast-feeding compared to formula and complementary feeding with meaningful differences concerning the recommended duration: for ES and HU the predominant advice was for exclusive breast-feeding for 6 months, for DE exclusive breast-feeding for 4–6 months and for UK and FI breast-feeding without further specification. In summary, statements relating to the programming of later obesity have been partially integrated into feeding information in five European countries. These countries have slightly different breastfeeding recommendations, but consistently refer to the preventive potential of

---

J. von Rosen-von Hoewel and B. Koletzko (✉)
Dr. von Hauner Children's Hospital, Ludwig-Maximilians-University, Munich, Germany
office.koletzko@med.uni-muenchen.de

K. Laitinen
Department of Paediatrics, University of Turku, Finland

E. Martin-Bautista and C. Campoy
Department of Paediatrics, University of Granada, Spain

V. Jakobik, T. Decsi
Department of Paediatrics, University of Pécs, Hungary

M.A. Schmid, J. Morgan, H. Gage, and M. Raats
Food, Consumer Behaviour and Health Research Centre, University of Surrey, Guildford, UK

B. Koletzko et al. (eds.), *Early Nutrition Programming and Health Outcomes in Later Life: Obesity and Beyond*,

breastfeeding in general. This is important as obesity and its resulting morbidity are of increasing public health concern in developed countries.

Keywords Breastfeeding • infant feeding • metabolic programming • nutrition programming

Abbreviations BF: breastfeeding; CF: complementary-feeding; CVD: cardiovascular diseases; GOV: government; IND: industry; MF: milk-feeding; PROF: professional associations; RCT: randomised controlled trials; SIG: special interest groups

1 Introduction

Childhood obesity is considered a global epidemic with worldwide prevalence and severity increasing at alarming rates (WHO 1998; Kopelman 2000; Popkin and Doak 1998) and it concerns affluent countries as well as countries in economic transition (Drewnowski and Popkin 1997; Martorell et al. 2000). Serious short and long term consequences of childhood obesity arise in terms of impairments of quality of life, performance and health. In addition to genetic predisposition and current lifestyle, nutritional programming is considered as an important risk factor for developing obesity. It is broadly defined as "either the induction, deletion, or impaired development of a permanent somatic structure or the setting of a physiological system by an early stimulus or insult operating at a sensitive period, resulting in long-term consequences for function" (Lucas 1991). Several indications exist that modification of infantile nutrition, such as promotion of breast feeding, may contribute to decreasing later obesity risk (Schack-Nielsen and Michaelsen 2006). The concept of early nutritional programming has recently gained wide acknowledgment among researchers (Koletzko 2006; Demmelmair et al. 2006), but there is little research on identifying the extent to which research conclusions and policy statements enter information provided to parents. The purpose of this study, conducted in five member states of the European Union (Finland, Germany, Hungary, Spain, and United Kingdom), is to determine the incorporation of information on the association between early diet and lifelong health, particularly concerning obesity, in leaflets and parenting magazine articles about infant feeding.

2 Material and Methods

2.1 Assessing Infant Feeding Leaflets

Between July and October 2005 a standardized web-based research procedure for assessing stand alone leaflets on infant nutrition referring to feeding of healthy infants aged

0–12 months was conducted in the five participating countries. Websites from national and regional government bodies, professional associations, special interest groups and the retailing and manufacturing industries were visited to locate materials covering the area of infant feeding using the key words: nutrition, diet, breastfeeding, bottle feeding, formula feeding, weaning, complementary feeding, infant feeding, and baby. Stand alone materials were either collected electronically or printed. Leaflets published after 2000 targeting parents were included. Materials targeting pregnancy, older children and health professionals or focusing on legal and practical aspects were excluded.

2.2 Assessing Articles and Notes in Parenting Magazines

The most popular monthly parenting magazine for each country was selected based on annual average circulation per issue figures. All 12 issues from 2005 were screened for articles and notes on infant feeding, i.e. about feeding of and nutrition for babies aged 0–12 months. Most popular was defined by the annual average circulation per issue.

2.3 Selection of Programming Statements

Materials were screened for statements on nutrition related programming in relation to milk and complementary feeding. As it was not expected to come across the term "programming" itself, all statements on regular feeding of a healthy infants resulting in certain health outcomes have been considered as relevant. Statements on non-nutritive or toxicological substances, non-nutrition related behaviour (e.g. smoking), as well as nutrient absorption and supplementation (e.g. of folic acid), non-metabolism related outcomes, and adverse health effects due to a special diet or severe malnutrition were excluded from the database.

Each statement was further characterized concerning the duration of health effect (not mentioned, short-term perspective, i.e. duration of effect less than 5 years, medium-term perspective, i.e. duration of effect from 5 to 15 years, and long-term perspective, i.e. duration of effect more than 15 years). The programming related feeding behaviour was coded as milk-feeding, complementary feeding, either period, or general statements on infant feeding. Milk-feeding was further divided into breastfeeding in general, exclusive breastfeeding without further specification, exclusive breastfeeding for 6 months, and formula feeding. It was noted whether a scientific reference was cited with the health outcome or not.

A final total of 638 valid programming statements, for example "breastfeeding helps to prevent obesity later in life", remained for analysis and were classified into 15 health outcome categories. All analyses were carried out with the software package SPSS (SPSS, 13.0, Chicago, IL, USA).

3 Results

In total, 130 leaflets published between 2000 and 2005 have been reviewed for analysis (Finland = 8, Germany = 14, Hungary = 38, Spain = 34, UK = 36). In summary, 76% of the leaflets contained programming statements, with considerable variation between the countries, ranging from 94% of the Spanish to 61% of the UK leaflets. The pattern of density of statements differed as well: in Germany there was an average of 9.6 statements per leaflet down to 1.1 statements per Finnish leaflet. About 20% of programming statements were based on a given reference. The 60 reviewed magazine issues contained 161 nutrition related articles and notes. In summary, 41% of the magazine contributions contained programming statements, with considerable variation between the countries ranging from 82% of the Spanish to 25% of the Finnish articles and notes. There was a country specific pattern concerning statements citing references, where Hungary, Spain, and the UK did not cite any references with the articles and notes, whereas 13% of the Finnish and 2% of the German magazine contributions referred to scientific literature.

Table 1 shows the order of the six most frequently mentioned health outcome categories per country. Allergy was the most frequent programming related health outcome in the UK (25.7%), Hungary (23.5%), and Germany (22.2%), whereas it was risk of infection in Spain (21.2%) and growth and development in Finland (18.4%). Obesity was mentioned in 8.5% (54/638) of the statements, thus in the cross-country comparison the fourth most frequent health outcome.

The majority of statements (68.2%, n = 435) did not refer to the duration of the programming related health effects, a further 18.2% (n = 122) referred to short- and 5.1% (n = 33) to medium-term duration. In total, only 8% of the statements referred to a long-term duration of programming effects, thus considering a lifelong approach. Among the obesity concerning statements a temporal prognosis was given in 39%, with 6% referring to short- (<5 years), 13% to medium- (5–15 years)

Table 1 Frequency of health outcomes associated with nutritional programming

Health outcome categories	UK		Finland		Germany		Hungary		Spain		All countries	
	n	%	n	%	n	%	n	%	n	%	n	%
Allergy	46	25.7	4	10.5	44	22.2	28	23.5	10	9.6	132	20.7
Risk of infection	41	22.9	3	7.9	13	6.6	20	16.8	22	21.2	99	15.5
Growth and development	10	5.6	7	18.4	34	17.2	9	7.6	13	12.5	73	11.4
Obesity	11	6.1	5	13.2	18	9.1	9	7.6	11	10.6	54	8.5
Risk of disease in general	19	10.6	3	7.9	10	5.1	9	7.6	10	9.6	51	8.0
Mental development	9	5.0	1	2.6	12	6.1	9	7.6	8	7.7	39	6.1
Other health outcomes	43	24.1	15	39.5	67	33.7	35	29.3	30	28.8	190	29.8

and 20% to long-term (>15 years) duration of effects. So obesity related statements were focused more than average on the intrinsic long-term perspective of programming compared to other surveyed health-outcomes. The major programming related behaviour concerned breast-feeding (47% all over, Hungary and Spain even 100%) compared to formula and complementary feeding with meaningful differences concerning the recommended duration: in Hungary and Spain the predominant advice was exclusive breast-feeding for 6 months, in Germany exclusive breast-feeding for 4–6 months and for Finland and the UK breast-feeding without further specification. The preventive aspect of breastfeeding towards later obesity was consistently included in the statements.

4 Discussion

The aim of this review was to survey to what extent the concept of early nutrition programming is being communicated to parents in written information. The focus was on leaflets, because of their important role as a source of advice for parents (DoH 2002). Magazines were included as they have also been recognized as having a practical impact on parental decision making (Foss and Southwell 2006).

The frequency of cited health outcomes showed a strong focus on diseases with onset close to the feeding period: the well-established associations between breast-feeding and infections (Howie et al. 1990; Golding et al. 1997) and breastfeeding or introduction of certain foods and allergies (Marini et al. 1996; Oddy et al. 2002) were responsible for 36.2% of all health outcomes. Obesity, which has already reached pandemic proportions in Europe (WHO 2003) was at least ranked fourth (8.5%) and particularly emphasized in Finland (13.2%) and Spain (10.6%).

Childhood obesity has short- and medium-term medical and psychosocial consequences in childhood and adolescence, as well as long-term effects that extend well into adulthood (Dietz 1998). This was reflected in the statements including references to the long-term duration of the health effects. It was a gratifying finding that breastfeeding was constantly recommended as preventive. Particularly in industrialized countries, promoting prolonged breast-feeding may help in decreasing the prevalence of obesity in childhood (von Kries et al.1999; Arenz et al. 2004). Although the underlying mechanisms remain to be elucidated, these findings emphasize the importance of early nutritional influences in addition to genetic disposition and current lifestyle.

To make informed choices and implement health improving feeding behaviour parents need to be able to acquire knowledge based on current scientific thinking. Therefore further emphasis should be placed on the dissemination of practical, achievable and realistic advice that clearly explains the possible long-term health benefits of appropriate feeding behaviour (Raats et al. 2005). The concept of early nutritional programming embodies great potential for the improvement of health and quality of life for future generations, which needs to be further communicated to parents.

5 Conclusions

In summary, statements relating to the programming of later obesity have been partially integrated into feeding information in five European countries, with the long-term perspective taken into account to a greater extent than for other health outcomes assessed in this survey. The five European countries included in the survey have slightly different breastfeeding recommendations, but consistently refer to the preventive potential of breastfeeding in general. This is important as obesity and its resulting morbidity are of increasing public health concern in developed countries.

Acknowledgements This study was supported by the European Project "Early Nutrition Programming-EARNEST" in the 6° Framework. N° FOOD-CT-2005-007036. Parts of this publication originate from the dissertation from J. v. Rosen-v. Hoewel.

References

Arenz S, Ruckerl R, Koletzko B, von Kries R (2004). Breast-feeding and childhood obesity – a systematic review. *Int J Obes Relat Metab Disord* **28**: 1247–1256.

Demmelmair H, von Rosen J, Koletzko B (2006, Aug). Long-term consequences of early nutrition. *Early Hum Dev* **82**(8): 567–574.

DoH (Department of Health) (2002, May). Infant feeding 2000: summary report. http://www.dh.gov.uk.

Dietz WH (1998). Health consequences of obesity in youth: childhood predictors of adult disease. *Pediatrics* **101**: 518–525.

Drewnowski A, Popkin BM (1997). The nutrition transition: new trends in the global diet. *Nutr Rev* **55**(2): 31–43.

Foss KA, Southwell BG (2006). Infant feeding and the media: the relationship between Parents' magazine content and breastfeeding, 1972–2000. *Int Breastfeed J* **1**: 10.

Golding J, Emmett PM, Rogers IS (1997, Oct 29). Gastroenteritis, diarrhoea and breast feeding. *Early Hum Dev* **49**(Suppl): 83–103.

Howie PW, Forsyth JS, Ogston SA, Clark A, Florey CD (1990). Protective effect of breastfeeding against infection. *Brit Med J* **300**: 11–16.

Koletzko B (2006). Long-term consequences of early feeding on later obesity risk. *Nestle Nutr Workshop Ser Pediatr Prog* **58**: 1–18.

Kopelman PG (2000). Obesity as a medical problem. *Nature* **404**(6778): 635–643.

Lucas A (1991). Programming by early nutrition in man: In: Bock GR, Whelan J (eds.), *The childhood environment and adult disease (CIBA Foundation Symposium 156)*. Wiley, Chichester, pp. 38–55.

Marini A, Agosti M, Motta G, Mosca F (1996, May). Effects of a dietary and environmental prevention programme on the incidence of allergic symptoms in high atopic risk infants: three years' follow-up. *Acta Paediatr Suppl* **414**: 1–21.

Martorell R, Khan LK, Hughes ML et al. (2000). Obesity in women from developing countries. *Eur J Clin Nutr* **54**(3): 247–252.

Oddy WH, Peat JK, de Klerk NH (2002). Maternal asthma, infant feeding, and the risk of asthma in childhood. *J Allergy Clin Immunol* **110**: 65–67.

Popkin BM, Doak CM. The obesity epidemic is a worldwide phenomenon. *Nutr Rev* **56**(4 Pt 1): 106–114.

Raats M, Poutanen K, Almeida M (2005). Consumer needs regarding dietetic products for pregnant and lactating women and for baby foods. *Adv Exp Med Biol* **569**: 120–126.

Schack-Nielsen L, Michaelsen KF (2006). Breast feeding and future health. *Curr Opin Clin Nutr Metab Care* **9**: 289–296.

von Kries R, Koletzko B, Sauerwald T et al. (1999). Breast feeding and obesity: cross sectional study. *BMJ* **319**(7203): 147–150.

World Health Organisation (1998). Obesity. Preventing and managing the global epidemic. Report of a WHO consultation on obesity. Geneva: World Health Organisation.

WHO (2003). Integrated prevention of non communicable disease. Draft global strategy on diet, physical activity and health. Document EB113/44. WHO.

Infant Feeding and the Concept of Early Nutrition Programming: A Comparison of Qualitative Data from Four European Countries

Martina A. Schmid, Julia von Rosen-von Hoewel, Elena Martin-Bautista, Éva Szabó, Cristina Campoy, Tamás Decsi, Jane Morgan, Heather Gage, Berthold Koletzko, and Monique Raats

Abstract The concept of early nutrition programming is appearing in policy documents, leaflets and magazine articles with different types of statements. However, the level of representation and influence of this concept is unknown in the area of infant nutrition. We established the degree of reflection and the impact of the concept of nutrition programming among the different government stakeholders of infant nutrition in four European countries. In each country, a list of stakeholders in the area of infant feeding was established and key persons responsible for the remit of infant nutrition were identified. We conducted standardised face-to-face or phone interviews from January 2006 to January 2007. The interview guide included questions about the concept of nutrition programming. All interviews were digitally recorded and qualitative data analysis was done using QRS NVivo V2. In total, we analyzed 17 interviews from government organizations in England (5 interviews), Germany (4 interviews), Hungary (3 interviews) and Spain (5 interviews). The concept of nutrition programming was recognized from 4/5 English and 3/4 German interviewees, whereby one organisation reflected the concept in their documents in both countries. In Hungary, 1/3 interviewees recognised the concept and reflected it in their documents. All interviewed Spanish governmental bodies (5/5) recognised the concept of nutrition programming and three of them reflected the concept in their documents. The concept of early nutrition programming was widely recognized among the key persons of government bodies in all four European countries. However, the concept was not necessarily represented in the produced documents.

M.A. Schmid, H. Gage, and M. Raats (✉)
Food, Consumer Behaviour and Health Research Centre, University of Surrey, Guildford, UK
m.raats@surrey.ac.uk

J. von Rosen-von Hoewel and B. Koletzko
Dr. von Hauner Children's Hospital, Ludwig-Maximilians-University, Munich, Germany

E. Martin-Bautista and C. Campoy
Department of Paediatrics, University of Granada, Spain

É. Szabó and T. Decsi
Department of Paediatrics, University of Pécs, Hungary

B. Koletzko et al. (eds.), *Early Nutrition Programming and Health Outcomes in Later Life: Obesity and Beyond*,

Keywords Infant feeding • metabolic programming • nutrition programming • nutrition policy

Abbreviations QRS: Qualitative Research System

1 Introduction

In the first stages of life, nutrition has a significant impact on the maintenance of lifelong health (Lucas 2005). The early diet can influence the neurological development (Dijck-Brouwer et al. 2005) and the development of several diseases, such as cardiovascular diseases (Reddy and Katan 2004), diabetes (Steyn et al. 2004), and certain types of cancer (Key et al. 2004). This concept is known as early nutrition programming or metabolic programming, which has gained broad recognition among researchers (Demmelmair et al. 2006), as evidence increasingly shows that breastfeeding (Koletzko 2006) and complementary feeding could have an impact on child development and long-term health (Lucas 2005; Demmelmair et al. 2006).

There is an increasing major public health interest about the concept of early nutrition programming and statements reflecting this concept are appearing in policy documents, leaflets and magazine articles targeting infant nutrition. However, the level of representation and influence of this concept among the different stakeholders in the area of infant feeding is unknown. The aim of this qualitative study was to establish the degree of reflection and the impact of the concept of early nutrition programming among key persons from government organisations and agencies with their remit of infant nutrition in England, Germany, Hungary and Spain.

2 Material and Methods

In 2006, a list of government stakeholder organisations or agencies in the area of infant feeding was established for England, Germany, Hungary and Spain. The key persons responsible for the remit of infant feeding were identified for each stakeholder and invited to participate in the study. The standardised interview guide included several questions about the concept of early nutrition programming. The following two questions were analysed in this paper: "*Have you come across the term or concept of nutrition programming?*" and "*How is the concept of nutrition programming reflected in your publications?*".

The face-to-face or phone interviews were conducted in the original language from January 2006 to January 2007 by the same four interviewers. The interviews were digitally recorded and qualitative data analysis was done using QRS NVivo V2.

2.1 Qualitative Data Analysis

As a first step the interview guide, including all questions, was developed in English and piloted. Then all interviews were conducted and transcribed in the original language in the four countries. A standardised coding tree in English was developed and used to identify the different statements made by the interviewees in regard to the concept of early nutrition programming in their original language. The identified statements were translated into English for further qualitative data analysis.

3 Results

In total, we interviewed 17 government organizations and agencies in England (5 interviews), Germany (4 interviews), Hungary (3 interviews) and Spain (5 interviews). Table 1 lists the government organizations and agencies with key persons who agreed to participate in the qualitative study.

England

Four interviewees from the five English government bodies with infant feeding in their remit recognized the concept of early nutrition programming. They quoted the following statements: "*Yes*", "*Well certainly not using that term*", and "*Nutrition programming, yes we certainly would use that, is that what you mean*".

One of the five interviewees stated with the following answer, that the concept was reflected in their documents: "One of the terms of references are to review the

Table 1 Interviewed government agencies in England, Germany, Hungary and Spain

Country	Government organisations and agencies
England	Department of Health
	National Health Service (NHS)
	Food Standards Agency
	National Institute of Clinical Excellence
	Scientific Advisory Committee on Nutrition (SACN)
Germany	Federal Institute for Risk Assessment
	Federal Ministry for Nutrition and Rural Area – Baden Würtenberg
	Bavarian Federal State Office for Health and Food Safety
	Bavarian Federal Ministry for Environment, Health and Consumer Protection
Hungary	National Institute for Food Safety and Nutrition
	National Institute for Child Health
	National Committee for Supporting Breastfeeding
Spain	Spanish Nutrition Society Scientific Research Council
	ESPGHAN Infant Nutrition Committee
	Spanish Paediatrics Association
	University of Granada
	University of Barcelona

evidence and the influence of maternal nutrition including growth and development so that will be incorporated within".

Germany

Three interviewees from the four German government agencies recognized the concept of early nutrition programming. They responded with the following statements: "*The idea of programming is that nutrition imprints the later activity of metabolic functions during a critical window*", "*the concept of programming sounds reasonable*", and "*the basis for the prevention of allergy and dietary intolerance is a health promoting nutrition*".

The concept of early nutrition programming was reflected in documents of one organisation. The interviewee answered as follows: "*Yes this is one of the pillars why policy are composed*".

Hungary

One key person of the three Hungarian interviews recognised the concept of early nutrition programming giving the following statement: "*Well this is what I was talking about*". In addition, the concept was reflected in their documents. The interviewee stated the following: "*Practically speaking I use it in my presentation and I try to attract attention to it*".

Spain

All five interviewees representing Spanish government organisations in the field of infant feeding recognised the concept of early nutrition programming. They gave the following answers: "*yes*", "*yes of course*", "*yes since some years ago*", and "*With this name not, but I imagine that you refer to the metabolism programming in the adult life while a good nutrition in the infancy*".

Three of the five interviewed key persons stated that their organisations were reflecting the concept in their documents as follows: "*We try to introduce the knowledge from our research projects in the formation of our future professionals*", "*there is only one publication about this theme*", and "*The results from our research, specially those related with metabolic alteration and gene expression in prepubertal obese children, are discussed based on this concept, it has not been yet reflected*".

4 Conclusions

In summary, the concept of early nutrition programming was widely recognized among the interviewed key persons from government organisations and agencies responsible for the remit of infant nutrition in England, Germany, Hungary and Spain. However, the concept of early nutrition programming was rarely integrated in the produced documents.

Acknowledgements This study was supported by the European Project "Early Nutrition Programming-EARNEST" in the 6° Framework. N° FOOD-CT-2005-007036.

References

Demmelmair H, von Rosen J, Koletzko B (2006, Aug). Long-term consequences of early nutrition. *Early Hum Dev* **82**(8):567–574.

Dijck-Brouwer DA, Hadders-Algra M, Bouwstra H, Decsi T, Boehm G, Martini IA, Boersma ER, Muskiet FA (2005, Jan). Lower fetal status of docosahexaenoic acid, arachidonic acid and essential fatty acids is associated with less favorable neonatal neurological condition. *Prostaglandins Leukot Essent Fatty Acids*, **72**(1):21–28.

Key YJ, Schatzkin A, Willett WC, Allen NE, Spencer EA, Travis RC (2004). Diet, nutrition and the prevention of cancer. *Public Health Nutr* **7**(1A):187–200.

Koletzko B (2006). Long-term consequences of early feeding on later obesity risk. *Nestle Nutr Workshop Ser Pediatr Prog* **58**:1–18.

Lucas A (2005, May). Long-term programming effects of early nutrition – implications for the preterm infant. *J Perinatol* **25**(Suppl 2):S2–S6.

Reddy KS, Katan MB (2004). Diet, nutrition and the prevention of hypertension and cardiovascular diseases. *Public Health Nutr* **7**(1A):167–186.

Steyn NP, Mann J, Bennet PH, Temple N, Zimmel P, Tuomilehto J et al. (2004). Diet, nutrition and the prevention of type 2 diabetes. *Public Health Nutr* **7**(1A):147–165.

What is the EARNEST Dissemination and Exploitation Consensus Panel (DECP)?

Margaret Ashwell and Anne de la Hunty

Abstract The Dissemination and Exploitation Consensus Panel (DECP) is a panel of experts drawn from areas with relevant expertise who advise the Early Nutrition Programming Project (EARNEST) on how the results from the project can best be disseminated and exploited and their uses maximised. They meet annually and have discussed how to communicate the results from the project more widely to health professionals. For example, what are the potential exploitable outcomes for different stakeholder groups are from the Childhood Obesity Project?

Keywords Dissemination • exploitation • health professionals

Abbreviations CHOP: Childhood Obesity Project; DECP: Dissemination and Exploitation Panel; EFSA: European Food Safety Authority; QC: quality control

1 Introduction

As well as scientific advisers, it is important for a large EC project like The Early Nutrition Programming Project (EARNEST) to have a panel of advisers to help spread the news about the project to the wider world and to help to suggest exploitable outcomes. We were therefore delighted to appoint such a group of experts (see Acknowledgments) and hold the first meeting of our Dissemination and Exploitation Consensus Panel (DECP) in Cambridge, UK in 2006 and the second in Prague in 2007.

M. Ashwell(✉) and A. de la Hunty
Ashwell Associates (Europe) Ltd. Ashwell, Herts., UK, SG7 5PZ
margaret@ashwell.uk.com

B. Koletzko et al. (eds.), *Early Nutrition Programming and Health Outcomes in Later Life: Obesity and Beyond*,

2 First Meeting of DECP

The panel became acquainted with the EARNEST project and met the main players who gave short summaries of their themes and outlined what were the possible exploitable outcomes from them. The Panel also discussed the ways in which they believed they could best help the project and what their role would be.

3 Second Meeting of DECP

The Panel discussed future dissemination opportunities and identified possible key routes to health professionals:

- The importance of getting onto the curriculum of different disciplines thus influencing the early education of young professionals
- The importance of training young scientists to act as unbiased translators of science for different target audiences
- The importance of getting Continuing Professional Development accreditation for our seminars and meetings

The need for Europe-wide dissemination activities was also discussed and the possibility of organising satellite meetings to national congresses was suggested as a way of penetrating at a deeper level in each country. "Direct to consumer" dissemination was identified as being important to create a market "pull". This might be fronted by a well-known celebrity/communicator who would increase interest in the subject.

Also at this meeting, Prof Berthold Koletzko gave a presentation on the Childhood Obesity Programme (CHOP) (see pages 15 – 29 for more details). This is one of the trials which is being followed up within the EARNEST project. Essentially, the trial showed that infants fed a formula which had a lower protein level from birth until 12 m of age were more similar, at 24 m, in weight for length to a reference group of breast fed infants than infants who had been fed a formula with higher protein levels.

The CHOP results were used as a case study to discuss exploitable opportunities which could then be a model to discuss further results emerging from the larger EARNEST project. The results were scrutinised using two different discussion frameworks:

(i) A Framework to discuss which exploitable outcomes from the CHOP project can be used by which stakeholder groups. The results of our discussions are summarised in Table 1 and show a very wide range of outcomes and possible use by stakeholder groups – as diverse as health professionals and health insurance companies.

(ii) Global Future Forecasting – The participants discussed a PESTLE analysis (political, economic, social, technological, legal and environmental) to give an indication of the drivers and trends which are likely to increase the importance of the CHOP results. These are summarised in Table 2. They are classified according to whether the drivers/trends will impact on the exploitable outcomes of the CHOP results in a positive, neutral or negative manner.

Table 1 Which stakeholder groups are likely recipients of the CHOP study results? How can they use them?

Government, policy makers	Health professionals	Food industry and trade associations	NGOs/charities and patient groups etc.	Health insurance companies	Popular media	Research community
Gives them options for making changes to Infant Formula Directive. Could decide to only permit formulae (infant and follow on) with lower protein levels or could recommend a narrower range of protein levels Can help them to calculate economic benefit of reduction in obesity from change in formula composition Gives more evidence if they decide to produce a policy on breastfeeding	Spread messages through the professional associations, e.g. Paediatricians, Midwives They could produce guidelines for lower protein load in first year Programming message important to encourage good eating patterns from early age Be aware of need to monitor growth of formula fed children particularly	Should be keen to exploit since cost neutral optionless protein reduces costs while more QC adds to them Good clear messages and consensus in the field to encourage companies to look at their portfolio of products Reassurance to companies now on safety aspects of lower protein They can be part of the solution to obesity problem and this is part of their due diligence	Message should be that breast is best, but if you don't breastfeed, pay particular attention to growth rates during first 2 years Some formulae (those with lower protein) are better than others – groups could recognise this and be willing to *promote* this message alongside the breastfeeding message	May want to support collection of more information on babies in this cohort to help them calculate risk There are ethical issues in health insurance E.g. insurance companies in Netherlands lower premium to functional food consumers (money back package) Health insurance recognises that people are healthier but that	A direct easy route to mothers is through websites, chat rooms Changing to a lower protein formula is a positive easily actionable step Should be presented as a solution not a problem – we must not make people anxious	Good studies – strong data so there should be many scientific publications from these results Some methodological advances should also be published e.g. the technique for 'blinding' the trial Shows it is possible to run harmonised studies and get valid results across five countries in EC projects But they lead to more and more questions: What has most influence? • Casein or what? • Branched chains amino acids?

(continued)

Matrix 1 (continued)

Government, policy makers	Health professionals	Food industry and trade associations	NGOs/charities and patient groups etc.	Health insurance companies	Popular media	Research community
		Common interest for the industry not a marketing gimmick Spur to industry to do more trials on other more novel components in formula, e.g. prebiotics		people also live longer. It is important to measure healthy years when calculating benefit		Does the effect persist into childhood and adulthood? Provides data for EFSA - advisers of the European Commission on infant nutrition Would the same effect be seen in undernourished populations?

Table 2 Possible drivers and trends which will impact upon the CHOP results (**positive**, neutral and negative)

Political	Economical	Social	Technological	Legal	Environmental
Further emphasis on strategies against obesity will help dissemination of these results	The increasing economic costs of obesity might encourage more exploitation of CHOP results. There will be a balance of the costs of living longer and the costs of ill health	**Increasing concern about rise in childhood obesity** **Men becoming more involved in child rearing because they can feed the baby. This would empower men and removes some of the guilt associated with bottle feeding**	**Improvements in food technology could mean that:** • **Industry can manipulate the amino acid content of formula more easily** • **Protein sources of infant formula can be produced to very high quality**	Ability to communicate to mothers becoming increasingly restricted due to concerns about formula advertising	Increasing concerns about environmental costs of industry activities. Are they carbon neutral? Will lower protein in infant formula result in less milk required for the production of the formula, and hence fewer cows, fewer fields, and less methane?
Greater investment in science will increase likelihood of funding of long term trials	**Increased European competitiveness in the world as a result of EC research should have positive effects on funding further EC research**	Consumers becoming more responsible and empowered for their own health – but do they want it? Personal happiness becoming more important – misery of fat children less acceptable but now not so uncommon Increasing migration means that we need to know if the effect is the same in undernourished children	• **More sophisticated whey fractions will be available for use in formula to make the amino acid profile even more similar to breast milk**	Increasing concerns that claims are not good ways of communicating with consumers	

4 Conclusions

Our DECP has already proved of immense value to the EARNEST project and we look forward to receiving even more advice from them as further results emerge from the project.

Acknowledgements We are very grateful to the panel for the time they have devoted to the EARNEST project. These are their names, countries and expertise: Chair: Prof. Dr. Hildegard Przyrembel (D-food policy); Members: Dr. Jean Michel Antoine (F-food industry); Dr. Heinz Bockler (D-infant food industry); Dr. Andrée Bronner (F-infant food industry trade association); Prof Michiel Korthals (NL-ethicist); Professor Frank Furedi (GB-social science), Dr. Lena Grimm (D-Intellectual Property rights) and Mrs. Carole Middleton (GB-Dietetics).

Subject Index

The manufacturer's authorised representative in the EU is Springer Nature Customer Service Centre GmbH, Europaplatz 3, 69115 Heidelberg, Germany. If you have any concerns regarding our products, please contact ProductSafety@springernature.com

Printed and bound by CPI Group (UK) Ltd, Croydon, CR0 4YY
30/09/2026
02225450-0020